Praise for
The **DNA** Way

*"Knowledge is power. Kashif reveals his health journey to help empower
you with the knowledge you need for your own longevity and vitality."*

— **Steven R. Gundry, M.D.**, *New York Times* best-selling author
of *The Plant Paradox*

*"I absolutely love how Kashif lays out a functional approach to our ge-
netics! When it comes to hormones, this perspective is massively needed!!
If you are looking to understand your genes and how to choose a lifestyle
that works with your genetics, then this is the book for you.
A game-changing resource that we have all been waiting for."*

— **Dr. Mindy Pelz**, fasting expert and *Wall Street Journal*
and national best-selling author

*"The insights that Kashif was able to deliver about the inner workings
of my brain and body were mind-blowing. It's like he accessed
my human instruction manual."*

— **Joe De Sena**, CEO and founder of Spartan Race

THE

DNA

WAY

Hay House Titles of Related Interest

YOU CAN HEAL YOUR LIFE, the movie,
starring Louise Hay & Friends
(available as an online streaming video)
www.hayhouse.com/louise-movie

THE SHIFT, the movie,
starring Dr. Wayne W. Dyer
(available as an online streaming video)
www.hayhouse.com/the-shift-movie

●●●●●●

*BECOMING SUPERNATURAL: How Common People
Are Doing the Uncommon,* by Dr. Joe Dispenza

*BEYOND LONGEVITY: A Proven Plan for Healing Faster,
Feeling Better, and Thriving at Any Age,* by Jason Prall

*GROW A NEW BODY: How Spirit and Power Plant Nutrients
Can Transform Your Health,* by Dr. Alberto Villoldo

*MEDICAL MEDIUM BRAIN SAVER: Answers to Brain
Inflammation, Mental Health, OCD, Brain Fog, Neurological
Symptoms, Addiction, Anxiety, Depression, Heavy Metals,
Epstein-Barr Virus, Seizures, Lyme, ADHD, Alzheimer's,
Autoimmune & Eating Disorders,* by Anthony William

All of the above are available at your local bookstore,
or may be ordered by visiting:

Hay House UK: www.hayhouse.co.uk
Hay House USA: www.hayhouse.com®
Hay House Australia: www.hayhouse.com.au
Hay House India: www.hayhouse.co.in

THE

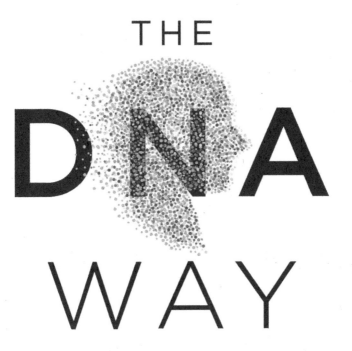

DNA

WAY

UNLOCK THE SECRETS OF YOUR GENES TO REVERSE DISEASE, SLOW AGEING AND ACHIEVE OPTIMAL WELLNESS

KASHIF KHAN

WITH ROD THORN

HAY
HOUSE

HAY HOUSE

Carlsbad, California • New York City
London • Sydney • New Delhi

Published in the United Kingdom by:
Hay House UK Ltd, The Sixth Floor, Watson House,
54 Baker Street, London W1U 7BU
Tel: +44 (0)20 3927 7290; Fax: +44 (0)20 3927 7291; www.hayhouse.co.uk

Published in the United States of America by:
Hay House Inc., PO Box 5100, Carlsbad, CA 92018-5100
Tel: (1) 760 431 7695 or (800) 654 5126
Fax: (1) 760 431 6948 or (800) 650 5115; www.hayhouse.com

Published in Australia by:
Hay House Australia Ltd, 18/36 Ralph St, Alexandria NSW 2015
Tel: (61) 2 9669 4299; Fax: (61) 2 9669 4144; www.hayhouse.com.au

Published in India by:
Hay House Publishers India, Muskaan Complex, Plot No.3, B-2,
Vasant Kunj, New Delhi 110 070
Tel: (91) 11 4176 1620; Fax: (91) 11 4176 1630; www.hayhouse.co.in

Text © Kashif Khan, 2023

Indexer: Joan Shapiro
Cover design: Jason Gabbert • *Interior design:* Nick C. Welch

The moral rights of the author have been asserted.

The information given in this book should not be treated as a substitute for professional medical advice; always consult a medical practitioner. Any use of information in this book is at the reader's discretion and risk. Neither the author nor the publisher can be held responsible for any loss, claim or damage arising out of the use, or misuse, of the suggestions made, the failure to take medical advice or for any material on third-party websites.

A catalogue record for this book is available from the British Library.

Tradepaper ISBN: 978-1-78817-896-9
E-book ISBN: 978-1-4019-7127-4
Audiobook ISBN: 978-1-4019-7128-1

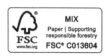

CONTENTS

FOREWORD

When I first met Kashif several years ago, a few things stood out.

The first was that Kashif is a natural storyteller. He speaks with a quiet directness that draws you in. He's passionate. He cares about what he's saying, and he says it with such clarity and earnestness that within seconds you start to care about it too.

At the time, the thing Kashif cared about—and convinced me to care about—was The DNA Company, which he had just co-founded. He was just getting it off the ground. As a founder of multiple companies, I knew what position Kashif was in. There's a reason most start-ups struggle. Starting a successful company is not for the faint of heart; it takes ambition, drive, vision, and work. And you have to care deeply. Kashif had some serious work ahead of him to achieve his worthy vision.

Most companies measure success by the money they make for their investors instead of by how they fulfill their mission or vision. From the start, Kashif has measured his success by the number of lives he can change. The DNA Company helps you take control of your genetics and use them to live better. You take a DNA test and get back a personalized lifestyle report—fitness recommendations, a diet plan, a supplement protocol, and potential health risks to avoid, tailored to your unique genetic code. It's the test that transformed my view of DNA tests as academically interesting but not actionable into the one I hold now, that a *functional* DNA test can help you know what kinds of control you have over your body.

In this book, Kashif goes a step further. He teaches you how to unlock the secrets of your genes to reverse disease, slow aging, and become the strongest version of yourself that you can be. As you read, you'll understand why Kashif has been so successful. He balances actionable, no-nonsense advice with easy-to-understand science and personal stories that hammer home his point: your health and performance are in your hands.

When you start to give your genetics what they want, you feel the difference in a visceral way. Your body and brain turn on. You wake up feeling good. You look better. You think with clarity and creativity that you didn't know you had. You unlock a level of performance that seems impossible, except to the few that dare to pursue it.

The pages that follow can save you hundreds of thousands of dollars and years of work. I don't say that lightly. In my early 20s I weighed 300 pounds. I was miserable. My brain didn't work. I had constant mood swings. I didn't feel a sense of purpose, which makes sense given that I had chronic fatigue syndrome and osteoarthritis. In short, my life sucked. I wasn't living in harmony with my genetics. I combed the ends of the earth looking for ways to fix my failing body and mind. I experimented with advanced yoga breathing exercises in India, meditation practices in Tibet, brain-wave monitoring, and cutting-edge neurofeedback. I tried a dozen diets, from raw vegan (which made things much worse) to Atkins (which made things a little bit better) to keto to eventually writing *The Bulletproof Diet*, a groundbreaking nutrition book that helped people lose 2 million pounds. I've spent 10 years and over $1 million figuring out what makes my body work and how I can change my diet and lifestyle to live a better life. And that was all without the benefits of knowing what to do with genetics.

Frankly, I wish I'd had this book 10 years ago. The knowledge in it is priceless. Kashif will teach you, step by step, how to leverage your genetics to achieve a level of potential you didn't know you could reach. He does so with wit, heart, humor, and clarity. Reading *The DNA Way* is a pleasure. Applying its lessons will change your life.

So take a deep breath, settle in, and get ready to learn the secrets of your DNA. Kashif will hand you the keys to living beyond what you thought was possible; what you do with that potential is up to you.

Dave Asprey
Founder, Bulletproof
CEO, Upgrade Labs, Danger Coffee, and 40 Years of Zen
New York Times best-selling author of *The Bulletproof Diet*,
Head Strong, *Fast This Way*, *Game Changers*, and *Super Human*
Victoria, BC
2022

INTRODUCTION

Yesterday I was clever, so I wanted to change the world.
Today I am wise, so I am changing myself.

— RUMI, 13TH-CENTURY SCHOLAR AND POET

It took me being lost at sea to find my purpose in life. That can happen when you're unmoored, buffeted by a raging wind and a roiling ocean, and your compass is broken.

And that's before I ever set foot on a boat.

When I think of the life journey I've been on, why I started The DNA Company, and why I'm writing this book, I'm reminded of the experience of Steven Callahan, a shipwreck survivor who spent 76 days adrift in a six-foot rubber life raft.

After enduring shark attacks and unrelenting storms and drifting directionless for 1,800 miles, all the while designing—in his head—a better survival vessel, the 30-year-old Callahan was rescued by fishermen. For the next 20 years he had many setbacks but worked steadily to bring his design to life, building an improved raft with a stiff shell, a removable canopy, and a sail. Besides actually building the raft he'd envisioned, he wanted to create something that could help others if they found themselves in a similar predicament.

Callahan was an accomplished sailor who had successfully crossed the Atlantic solo before getting lost at sea, and he had used his near-death experience to serve as an advisor on the film *Life of Pi*. If you're not familiar with this film, a young Indian boy is stranded at sea on a lifeboat, his only companion a tiger. The tiger—whether it's a real animal or a figment of the boy's imagination is up to the viewer—represents the intrinsic quality that makes living organisms do whatever is necessary to survive.

From my position at The DNA Company, I think of that intrinsic quality in terms of DNA—the unchanging language of life. At the same time, I know that a person's DNA is not their destiny. The choices people make about their nutrition and lifestyle and environment impact their health and survival as living organisms. This is one of the meanings I took away from the film, and Callahan, with his epic experience, was an ideal advisor for me.

Despite all that he'd accomplished, Callahan still considered his life to be largely unsuccessful. However, like the rogue whale that sank his sailboat, something unexpected happened—in the process of designing a vessel that could help others, he himself became a better person.

In my case, although I was only metaphorically lost at sea, and was already financially quite successful, the realization that my life was a wreck did begin on the ocean.

I was in my mid-30s and had gone out on a boat with some friends. What we were celebrating, I can't remember—by itself, that says a lot about me. I do know there was food and music and jokes and laughing and general hilarity.

What I will never forget is looking at a picture one of my friends sent me a couple of weeks after that day on the boat. I was shocked. I wasn't obese, but I was overweight. I was still a young man, but my skin wasn't healthy; I had ugly red patches of itchy, burning eczema on several parts of my body. I had poor posture, and I seemed to have no energy. My eyes were heavy and had dark circles under them. I knew that behind those eyes I was suffering from intense migraines. Most concerning was that the person I was looking at in the photo did not have any joy. Not just that day, but every day. I may have been laughing and seeming to have a good time, but I was playing a part I thought I was supposed to play—that of a successful entrepreneur living it up, celebrating some victory, a master of the universe. But I felt empty inside. I was figuratively adrift, and I knew it. What made the moment more haunting was the song that was playing in my head as I looked at the photo, "Take a Picture" by Filter.

The photo I was holding told a story. And if I didn't make some changes in how I was living, that story would not end well. I knew this because I'd experienced it in my own family.

My father, who died when he was only 71, had a tough life. He was from Shimla, which is in northern India and is the capital and the largest city in the state of Himachal Pradesh. During the partition era of India and Pakistan, he and his family fled the country on a train, first to the port city of Karachi, in Pakistan, then to Singapore, and finally to British Columbia in Canada—a nearly 13,000-mile ordeal. When they arrived, his two brothers stayed in Vancouver, one becoming a real estate investor, the other opening a textile business. My father went to Kelowna, about a four-hour drive from Vancouver, where he worked in a sawmill for a while and then on a potato farm, sending money back to Vancouver to try to do his part to support the family. His six brothers and two sisters used that money to start a business importing goods.

By the time my sister and I were born in Victoria, she in 1977 and me in 1979, we were very poor, and my father was constantly sick with diabetes, heart disease, and other ailments. His brothers resented him because he was only able to work intermittently and couldn't contribute much. When we moved from Victoria to Vancouver, we lived in a 600-square-foot apartment, my parents in one bedroom, my sister and me in the other. When we got older my parents slept in the living room so my sister and I could have our own rooms. They slept on a mattress they'd sawed in half, storing the pieces behind the couches until it was time to bring them back out at night. We often had to go without food and never had friends come to the apartment because we were embarrassed by our living conditions. When I did get any birthday presents from relatives, I had to sell them and use the money to buy school supplies.

My father was trying to make a go of it by buying old cars, then fixing and selling them. He had built up some inventory and was doing okay until a fire broke out and destroyed all his cars, causing him to lose everything. Devastated, with his health worsening, he turned to his best friend, a pharmacist, who gave him supplements to sell. Soon, he began taking the supplements himself, thinking they might help his diabetes and heart disease. What he didn't know was that they contained a potentially dangerous blood thinner. One day, not long after he started the supplements, while he was talking with someone, he had a brain aneurysm because of the blood thinner and dropped dead on the spot.

I didn't know it then, but it might have all been prevented if my grandparents had understood my father's DNA. If they had known he had a genetic predisposition to diabetes and heart disease, they could have fed him different foods and steered him to make better lifestyle choices as he got older. If only my father had known how he would react to the supplements he was taking—which a study of his DNA would have revealed—he wouldn't have taken them.

If only.

Of course, none of that was on my mind when I was suddenly thrust into the role of man of the house—and breadwinner—at the age of 17. My mother was also in poor health due to hormone issues, and my sister, who had suffered brain damage during birth, couldn't really do much to bring in money. I had some skills, I was intelligent, and I was driven to make something of myself and take care of the family. So, when the reality of my instant adulthood arrived in the form of Visa calling in the $7,000 debt my father had incurred trying to build his car business, I had to make some tough choices.

For instance, although I'd been accepted to study mechanical engineering at a university, I couldn't attend. My high school teammates and I—my high school had a university-grade technical lab—entered a competition to see who could build the electric car that would go the farthest on a single charge. We won, beating even the university students, and people were calling us "whiz kids." But with the weight of immediate financial responsibility for my family bearing down on me, my university studies were not to be.

I started working with my uncle in his textile business and quickly discovered he was an alcoholic. As he grew more unstable and his business and life unraveled, I was left to pick up the threads. By the time I was 19 years old, I was running his business. If you know anyone who's 19, or you remember being 19 yourself, that is not a winning strategy. But I kept at it.

Another uncle, who was doing well in real estate, loaned me $5,000 to make a down payment on a house so I could move my mother and sister and me out of our tiny apartment. I bought one for $214,000, lived in part of it, and rented the rest out. Even in my living arrangement I was thinking about how to bring in money.

After a few years of working in the textile business and renting out our house, I'd had enough. All I'd known while living in Vancouver was an extended family that had serious problems—alcoholism and addiction, bipolar disorder, suicide, heart disease, diabetes, and multiple other physical and mental illnesses. I wanted and needed a fresh start.

One of my cousins had started a business in Toronto importing and selling expensive jewelry and gems. So I took my mother and sister, moved to Toronto, and joined him. For a while we did well. But after building the business by putting in 20 hours a day every day for five years, I discovered my cousin was operating with some unsavory characters and was also engaging in business practices that were, if not illegal, unethical. To be blunt, he was ripping people off, including me. Rather than go through a lengthy legal battle to regain the millions of dollars he'd stolen from me, I decided to cut my losses, walk away, and start my own jewelry and luxury import business.

One of my suppliers, who was five doors away from my office, heard what I was doing, said he had some inventory I could sell, and asked if I wanted to partner with him. I did, and in our first year together we increased revenue by 3,000 percent. From there, I was a man on fire. I bought and sold unbelievable gems such as a rare $10 million flawless 7.5-carat fancy blue diamond, a 30-carat yellow diamond, and many others. I held a $20 million auction at the Royal Ontario Museum. I branched out, starting other companies in public relations, investments, and luxury goods. I'd gone from a 600-square-foot apartment to real wealth by my mid-30s. And still it wasn't enough. It was . . . never . . . enough.

Until I saw the picture of myself on that boat. And I took a hard look at my life.

I realized I had been working nonstop, building successful entrepreneurial ventures, since I was 19 years old. I was making a lot of money, but besides my family, whom I felt obligated to support, what was I doing for other people besides also making them rich? I had lived the life of an immigrant—work like a dog, take care of your family, nothing else matters—but that was supposed to be the narrative of my father and his generation, not mine. Spirituality, friendships, health, family: all were put to the side to focus on work. And boy, did they all suffer.

My Wake-Up Call

I got migraines and brain fog so extreme I had to leave work and go home to sleep. I developed bad flareups of eczema, hives, rashes, and other skin conditions. I became depressed and even claustrophobic. MRIs, CT scans, and other tests showed early signs of inflammation and the beginning stages of chronic disease. The doctors prescribed some pills and creams and ointments and said, "Classic case of stress. Nothing to worry about it. We'll keep an eye on it."

It was then that a series of events happened to change my life. At first, I didn't see any connection. But in retrospect, they happened exactly as they were supposed to.

In one instance, I was talking with two of my luxury goods customers, both billionaires, one of whom ran a hedge fund and bought a $2 million diamond off me, the other who ran a gold mining company and was in the middle of a $100 million project. For some reason, instead of thinking how I could get them to spend more of their money with me, I thought, *Neither of these guys is any smarter than I am, and they are passionate about what they do. Why can't I have that?* And by that I did not mean financial success. I meant passion. A sense of purpose. A drive to make a big impact by helping other people. There was nothing to do with the thought but notice it and sit with it. Or, as the doctor said, "Keep an eye on it."

In another instance, I met and became friends with a pharmacologist named Harris Khan—we're not related; there are more than 23 million people in the world named Khan. When I told Harris what I was going through, he warned me about being in the early stages of chronic disease and suggested I take some supplements to address my inflammation. The knowledge that my father had taken the same route and passed away as a result was not lost on me. Neither was the idea that I could end up like him, with chronic diseases, even without taking a supplement. I told Harris about my father and I having this parallel experience, and he planted the thought that perhaps my genetics had something to do with my issues. To that end, I became a self-taught student of genetics. And I convinced Harris to start The DNA Company with me.

Then I met Dr. Mansoor Mohammed, who was like an entire library of books and university classes about genetics rolled into one person. There's no other way to say it. One of only a few people in the world who can read the human genome, he began studying for his Ph.D. when he was just 15 years old. That means when I was playing baseball, skiing, and taking tae kwon do, he was busy being a genius. I was introduced to Mansoor, who was running a clinical genomics practice in Toronto, by Bryce Wylde, a clinician and fellow DNA Company founder who said I was lucky to have the most knowledgeable man in functional genomics right in my backyard. I listened as Mansoor spoke about how genomics is much more involved than we see on television, how it impacts everything in our lives, and how most of the health care issues we deal with could be prevented if we only knew our DNA. I was mesmerized. Not only was I intellectually curious about what he was saying, I was personally motivated because of my health.

With those men as my catalyst, I embarked on an even more ambitious course of learning about genetics. I wanted to learn as much as I could as fast as I could. I read articles and studies. Subscribed to scientific journals. Went to conferences. Talked to experts. Even took classes on genetics at Harvard University.

Most important, I got my genetics tested. I looked back at my youth and my upbringing and asked: Could genetics be responsible for the addiction and achievement and illness and premature aging that was all around me and within me?

What I found was startling. Dopamine is the pleasure or reward-seeking neurochemical. It's the thing that gives you that feeling of WOW when you bite into a tasty pizza. It's responsible for the hit you get when you achieve something. And there's an actual gene called DRD2 that determines to what degree you bind that dopamine, meaning to what degree you experience that pleasure. I happen to have a version of DRD2 that has the lowest receptor density, so I don't feel things deeply. On top of that, I have an ultra-fast version of a gene called COMT, which makes the protein to clear the dopamine and bring the mind back to normal. Together, these two genes mean I hardly feel pleasure or reward, and once I do, I'm already clearing the experience before I'm even done with it. Then, I want that "hit" again. And again. And again. Ad infinitum.

Now, there are three possible outcomes for somebody like me. Depression, because you don't get that sense of pleasure and satisfaction. Addiction, because you constantly seek that third-party sense of pleasure. And achievement, because you filter your experience through reward as opposed to pleasure, and you keep challenging yourself. Whatever you did yesterday isn't good enough anymore. That's a tough formula to live by.

I got blessed, in one respect, that I went down the path of achievement through entrepreneurialism. But others in my family with the exact same genetic makeup went down different paths. They turned to alcohol for their dopamine hit.

Through this knowledge, I learned that until you truly understand the genetics of your mind, you can't really understand who you are or how you perceive the world around you. And personalizing that helps you get through whatever it is you're trying to challenge yourself with, or whatever it is that's challenging you.

When I took an even deeper dive into my genes, I found them to be an uncanny match for my personality and business acumen. For instance, I have a strong ability to multitask and a high tolerance for risk and danger, all of which shows up in my genetic profile. In addition, my genes reveal a reduced ability to detoxify pollutants, fumes, environmental chemicals, and pesticides. Despite my steely executive functioning, I am much more chemically sensitive than my colleagues.

I experienced the effects of my reduced detoxification ability when we were building The DNA Company's state-of-the-art facility. When I visited the construction site while industrial floor sealants were still being applied, I developed a severe eczema reaction within hours of exposure. After I stayed away from the facility for two weeks, my eczema flare had all but disappeared. When I returned to the construction site, my condition came right back. The reason? My innate, inherited detoxification pathways could not handle this overload. To defend me against such toxins, my colleagues at The DNA Company developed a personalized supplement for me that included the correct dose of N-acetylcysteine (NAC), selenium, milk thistle, and alpha-lipoic acid (ALA). These nutrients enhance my suboptimal detoxification pathway and enable my body to deal with pollutants and chemicals while reducing my risk of long-term illness.

Now seeing my health through a new lens, I dove even deeper and started to see the genetic pathways that led to my father's early passing when I was only 17 years old. I found the root cause for the multiple battles with addiction among his uncles and cousins. I understood why my mother stopped working in her 40s from hormonal issues that eventually led to surgery. And above all I learned that, with my DNA decoded, chronic disease was now a choice.

I never thought that I would be in better shape in my 40s than in my 20s. But I am. I started with easy fixes like what I was designed to eat and understanding what things were making me sick. I changed my fitness routine to lean more heavily on strength training, because the typical cardiovascular exercise I was doing was causing more harm than good. I paid attention to the toxins in my environment. I got more sleep, including during the day in naps, a previously unimaginable thought. Finally, I incorporated spirituality into my life, joining a community that prays together and seeks to help others in need. It was no accident that shortly after I joined the congregation, a guest speaker said, "We have a disease of worshipping money and achievement in our community instead of love and service."

Within a few weeks of making these changes, I looked and felt different.

I have since continued my quest and optimized my cellular systems to address concerns that could arise from my genetic profile, such as prostate health, cardiovascular disease, diabetes, and depression. Studying my DNA and taking appropriate actions has not only given me a new view of the future but has also told me what choices to make to have the best results. So much so that now, I no longer fear old age.

In fact, I came to my ultimate realization: success is not about adding sick years to your life, but about adding healthy life to your years—and more years.

Finally, I was so affected by everything I'd learned that I raised $3 million, bought Mansoor's research lab, and asked Harris Khan and Mansoor to join me in starting The DNA Company. I'd changed myself, and now I wanted to change the world.

Big talk from a little guy like me, right? Well, a couple of years ago I was in a museum with my family and saw a painting on the wall that looked exactly like the picture I use on my WhatsApp profile—an old guy in a turban smoking shisha. I thought, *What a coincidence.* When I showed the profile picture to my mother and she looked at the painting of the man and the description next to it, which said he was the 18th-century ruler of what is now modern-day Afghanistan, she casually said, "What do you know? That's your tenth-generation grandfather."

It turns out studying my DNA told me not only about my health but about the character I've inherited. The king of Kabul had a modest upbringing and was known for being generous, modest, and compassionate even after he rose to power. Unlike other rulers of the period who rose to fame because of their military prowess, cruelty, and authoritarianism, he was a benevolent man who was genuinely concerned with the welfare of his people. His unusual mixture of vitality, ambition, rationality, and goodwill created a balanced and virtuous state in a notably fierce and anarchic century. To that end, while he could have been called "king," he preferred the less pretentious title of "representative of the people." Finally, I learned I share a bit of a rebellious streak with the monarch— just as he did not seek approval to implement his reforms from any religious authority, I do not seek approval from any medical or pharmaceutical authority to implement my ideas about reversing disease, aging more slowly, and optimizing performance.

As "representatives of the people," my colleagues and I want to change the world one person at a time, starting with you.

How to Use this Book

Over the next 10 chapters I will discuss how Western society's current health care approach isn't working and why using DNA to personalize health care is the best way to prevent and reverse chronic disease, slow the aging process, and achieve optimal wellness.

I'll give an easy-to-understand primer on what genetics is and how the various elements of the human genome all work together.

Because bodies consist of interconnected and interdependent systems, I'll discuss how people often have more than one health issue at the same time.

I'll examine what it means to be a "biomedical explorer" and educate yourself on the aspects of science that can help you live a life full of health and vitality. I'll also talk about some of the people who are inspiring me on my journey and what they're doing.

I'll illustrate how the interdependency of genetics, nutrition, lifestyle, and the environment manifested in a personal way, through a health care crisis with my niece—a crisis that helped me change the course of my company and my personal mission.

I'll talk about how The DNA Company has studied the genomes of more than 7,000 people to date, analyzed their biochemistry at a cellular level, and determined how their choices—nutritional, environmental, lifestyle—interact with their DNA to impact their health. I'll discuss how we take each patient's data and produce individualized reports that are curated into seven core bodily systems: cardiovascular, fitness, diet, sleep, mood and behavior, immunity and detox, and longevity. I will also cover an approach we take that is critical to success; we don't just dump confusing, scary, and nonactionable data on people. Instead, we provide them with a coaching concierge to help them interpret the information and take the appropriate actions.

I'm going to take a unique approach to talking about all of these things—I'm going to make my own personal DNA test results public. In so doing, I'll describe how those results impact each of my seven core bodily systems, as well as outline recommendations that have helped me prevent or reverse illness, slow down the aging process, and optimize my performance. In essence, I will act as my own scientific case study. I can't say each of you should follow the recommendations that I have—after all, the recommendations are made based on the specific results of DNA tests, whether they're performed by my company or by another gene-testing company. But at least you'll get an idea of how the testing and results have impacted me.

Considering the rapid advances being made in gene editing, I will include a section that discusses the technical barriers and ethical concerns in using the method, which scientists are currently implementing to change the DNA of organisms such as plants, bacteria, and animals, to potentially treat genomic diseases in humans like cystic fibrosis and cancer. The science to do this on a reliable basis is not there yet, but it is coming quickly.

In my conclusion, I'll update you on the progress my niece and I are making, I'll ask you to imagine a world that is free from chronic disease, and I'll inspire you to act.

Part One

THE
SITUATION

Chapter 1

MEDICAL WHAC-A-MOLE

America's health care system is neither healthy, caring, nor a system.

— Walter Cronkite, journalist and author

Remember Whac-A-Mole? You probably played the game at arcades and carnivals, as I did, when you were a kid.

If you're not familiar with the game, here's how it works: You stand in front of a machine that is roughly waist or chest high. The machine has a play area with five holes, an electronic scoring display, and a large rubber mallet on a rope. At random times, small plastic moles pop up from the holes and go back down. As play goes on the speed gradually increases. Your task is to whack each mole before it recedes back into its hole.

It took me a while to figure out that the faster I whacked the moles, the higher my score would be. I was young, and I didn't understand why the moles kept popping up after I whacked them with the mallet. I didn't care so much about the score; I simply wanted the moles to stop popping up. I wanted to see a result from my action. And I never did because there were *always moles still sticking up at the end of the game.*

The game was tailor-made to take advantage of someone with my brain chemistry.

Because I had versions of the DRD2 and MAO genes that didn't do a good job of binding dopamine—the hormone that enables you to experience pleasure, satisfaction, and motivation—I didn't feel things deeply. In addition, my COMT gene, which cleared the dopamine, was lightning fast. Taken together, this meant I hardly felt anything when I whacked a mole, and when I did, the feeling was gone almost instantly. If I didn't want to turn into an irrational little maniac or crash emotionally, I had to quickly replenish my dopamine and keep replenishing it. In other words, I had to keep dumping quarters into the game and playing. Because I am also genetically wired to be a problem solver, this fruitless behavior was incredibly frustrating, and costly, as I could not afford to put even one quarter in.

Today, the United States is playing medical Whac-A-Mole. So is most of Western society, but it is particularly acute in the U.S.

In the U.S., we don't have a health care system. We have a sick care system—one that relies on expensive drugs and surgeries to manage symptoms after they pop up instead of getting at their root causes, thus ensuring a continual supply of symptoms to treat. This is financially lucrative for the health care industrial complex, but it does little for the patients who are its customers.

There are many things we should be doing. We should be helping citizens understand how their DNA—their own personal instruction manual—can help them prevent and reverse disease, slow the aging process, and be their best. We should be proactively teaching them how their nutritional, lifestyle, and environmental choices interact with their unique genetics to affect their lives, for better or worse. And we should be giving them the tools to partner with their clinicians to take charge of their own health and well-being, so they can live life to their fullest potential.

Instead, what we are doing is inefficient, ineffective, and ruinously expensive.

We know that firsthand because we feel it in our bank accounts and in our bodies. We are spending more, and we are getting sicker.

The Cost of Illness

While we have become experts in healing broken bones, performing surgeries, and treating terminal diseases, according to the Centers for Disease Control and Prevention (CDC), acute medical issues represent only about 10 percent of health care spending in the U.S. The other 90 percent is spent on putting temporary bandages on chronic, preventable, and reversable illnesses like high blood pressure, high cholesterol, type 2 diabetes, depression, anxiety, obesity, eating disorders, sleep disorders, immune system disorders, and more.

How much are we spending?

According to the American Medical Association and the Centers for Medicare and Medicaid Services (CMS), in the U.S. in 2020, national spending on health care surpassed $4 trillion ($4.125 trillion) for the first time. That's a 9.7 percent increase over 2019, and a record 19.7 percent of the U.S. gross domestic product.

Think I'm being an alarmist? That those numbers must be inflated because of COVID-19? They are, but only partially—about 36 percent of the increase in federal expenditures for health care were due to the COVID-19 pandemic.

This trend of soaring health care costs has been going on for at least the last 50 years. For perspective, in 1972, the total amount the U.S. spent on health care was $83.4 *billion*. By 2026, estimates say, it will reach $5.7 *trillion*. By 2028, $6.2 trillion.

Numbers that big can seem abstract. Like they don't apply to you. If you feel that way, consider this: in 2020, every individual spent $12,530—an 9.7 percent increase over the previous year—on health care. For the average American family, the amount is close to $30,000. Not many people have that kind of money laying around.

With medical expenses that high, it's not surprising that people and families are feeling financial stress. To that end, a new study by academic researchers from Harvard University, Hunter College, Indiana University, the University of Idaho, and the University of Illinois found that 66.5 percent of all bankruptcies are tied to medical issues—either because of high costs for care or time out of work. An estimated 530,000 families file for bankruptcy each year because of medical issues and bills, researchers found.

Perhaps you think the Affordable Care Act solved that problem because more people were able to become insured? While it is good that more people have coverage, the quality of their health care insurance has not been up to the task of reducing their costs. In fact, according to the *American Journal of Public Health*, which published the academic research I've just cited, the number of debtors who said medical issues were a contributing reason for their bankruptcy *increased* slightly after the law's implementation—67.5 percent in the three years following the law's adoption versus 65.5 percent prior.

On what are the U.S. and its citizens spending all that money?

It's a complex mix of hospital visits, health care administration, diagnostic tests, and more. But let's look at the one expenditure that directly hits the bank accounts of most citizens—prescription drugs.

In the United States, the total amount of money spent on medicines in 2020 reached approximately $539 billion. Out of that number, CMS reported retail prescription drug expenditures came to some $348.4 billion. For perspective, in 1960, that number was $2.7 billion. By 1970, it was more than double, at $5.5 billion.

Who is taking all of these medications, and for what? About 66 percent of U.S. adults take prescription drugs. About 46 percent of U.S. adults have taken a prescription drug in the past 30 days. If we look at similar countries, we see that in the United Kingdom, more than 26 percent of adults take prescription medications, about 35 percent of Australians take prescription medicine daily, and about 65 percent of Canadians ages 40 to 79 take one or more prescription drugs.

Prescription drug use tends to increase with age. According to the National Health and Nutrition Examination Survey of 2015–2016, 18 percent of children ages 0 to 11 years old reportedly used prescription drugs in the past 30 days. For adolescents ages 12 to 19 years old, the number is 27 percent. For adults ages 20 to 59 years old, it's 47 percent. And about 85 percent of adults ages 60 or older reportedly used prescription drugs in the past 30 days.

The CDC reports that every year in the U.S., pharmacists fill more than 4 billion prescriptions, a number that is expected to substantially increase by 2024. Data suggests, among those Americans who take prescription medications, the average number they take is four, with more than 131 million taking at least one.

The therapeutic areas where spending is the greatest are diabetes, cancer, autoimmune diseases, and respiratory diseases. Based on the number of prescriptions filled, antihypertensives, pain relievers, and mental health drugs are the leading classes.

The coronavirus pandemic has increased prescription drug use and impacted the way people get their medications. In the past year, there were increases in prescription fills among many drugs, especially those that were thought to treat COVID-19, as well as supplements, antidepressants, and stimulants for attention deficit hyperactivity disorder (ADHD).

You can probably see yourself or someone you know in one of these statistics. In fact, given how prevalent prescription medication use is, you may know someone in every one of them.

I am not anti–prescription drugs; they help people all around the world treat medical conditions. But they can also cause harm if they're misused. According to the American Psychological Association, the misuse of opioid pain relievers and stimulants has also risen during the pandemic as people attempt to cope with conditions like anxiety and depression. And that's on top of this startling fact cited by the National Survey on Drug Use and Health: prescription drug misuse has increased by 250 percent over 20 years.

The Power of DNA

The truth is, even if we're using medications for good reasons, I am certain we could be taking a lot less of them if we understood what our DNA is telling us and how our choices—lifestyle, nutrition, and environment—impact our health and well-being. In my case, before I took charge of my own health, I was using at least five or six different medications to treat my various ailments. In that regard, my "American dream" was right on track: by age 50, I would most likely be diagnosed with a chronic disease; by age 60, I'd have two, and I'd take for granted that the last 15 years of my life would be spent receiving high-priced medical treatment.

As I said earlier, we have a health care system that promises us the best acute care any civilization has ever offered. However, that same toolkit is used for chronic conditions. We wait for the problem and then treat it, but we never ask why it happened in the first place. Chronic conditions don't start on the day you find them. They require 7, 10, 15 years of us making the wrong choices, those misaligned with our genetic code, for us to eventually get sick.

That's how I knew what was in store for me, and where you may be headed if you don't act now.

Canaries in the Coal Mine

By now, the story of coal miners using canaries as early warning systems has become a cliché, a metaphor for something going terribly wrong. Although the practice ended in 1986 when British legislators gave miners a year to replace the last 200 canaries still in use (American and Canadian miners also used them) with electronic carbon monoxide sensors, the metaphor fits for our current health care approach.

In the course of their work coal miners encounter continual threats to their lives: being buried alive in cave-ins, being blown up in firedamp and coal dust explosions, being trapped by fires, and breathing deadly gases like carbon monoxide. The gas is insidious because it can't be smelled or seen, and it is deadly because it displaces oxygen molecules from the bloodstream so they can no longer get to vital tissues and organs. Carbon monoxide poisoning sneaks up on you too, starting with a slight headache, shortness of breath, and a feeling of light-headedness before turning fatal.

What do canaries have to do with coal mining?

The notion of using canaries came from John Scott Haldane, a Scottish physician and physiologist, in 1911. His discoveries about the human body and the nature of gases, particularly when investigating mining explosions, caused him to suggest using the birds to detect carbon monoxide. If the canary became sick or keeled over, it was time for the miners to get out.

Why canaries? It turns out they, like other birds, are considerably more sensitive to airborne toxins than humans are. Since birds take in an extraordinary amount of oxygen when they inhale *and* exhale—stored in sacs to enable them to quickly fly to great heights that would make humans sick—they also get an extra dose of whatever poisons might be in that air. By putting the vulnerable birds in harm's way, miners got their early-warning system.

Pity the canaries. I've read that the miners thought of them as pets, whistling to the birds and coaxing them as they worked. And after explosions did occur, they carried the birds in special cages designed to revive them when they reached the surface. But none of that makes me feel any better about all the innocent and defenseless canaries that were sacrificed on the way to enriching the owners of the mines in which they fluttered and sputtered.

The children of today are the canaries of yesterday. While sacrificing canaries may have been a practical reality to keep miners safe 110 years ago, there is no reason—given everything we now know about genetics—for our unwitting children to be early-warning systems for our poor health care system. And they are.

Let me tell you how I came to this conclusion.

As I scanned the news one morning in the fall of 2020, I winced at the *Toronto Star* headline: "The Kids Are in Crisis—and COVID-19 Is Making It Worse. In Canada, Deteriorating Youth Mental Health Is Leaving a Generation in Distress."

Like most parents, I often read news that concerns me. And as the CEO of The DNA Company, I help people of all ages and from all walks of life—from professional athletes, to people who want to perform more effectively at work, to children—use advancements in genetics and biotechnology to live healthier and more satisfying lives. In the course of my work, I've dealt with childhood learning disabilities, concussions, Lyme disease, autism, ADHD, dysfunctional hormones, and many other issues, including the mental health crisis cited in the *Toronto Star* headline.

But it was a call from my mother that made my knees buckle.

"Kashif, come quick!"

"What happened?" I said. "Are you all right?"

"Not me. Nur!" she yelled. "It's an emergency!"

Nur is my 14-year-old niece, my sister's daughter, who lives at my mother's house. My sister was out of town.

"Nur is on the floor," my mother said. "She's got her hands to her throat!"

"Is she choking?"

"I don't know! She says she can't breathe!"

I'd shut my laptop and was getting ready to dash out my office door.

"She *says* she can't breathe?" I slowed down. "She can talk?"

"Yes, yes!" she said. "She's crying and sweating and shaking."

I rushed home, and as any responsible adults would do, my mother and I took my niece to the hospital. The doctor who saw her for about 15 minutes said, "Classic anxiety attack. Nothing to worry about," and sent us on our way.

It happened again a month later when she passed out and fell in my mother's kitchen, this time physically injuring herself because she hit her head on the counter on the way down. Again, I got the call and took her to the hospital.

This time I spent the entire day in the hospital while they took blood samples and X-rays and CT scans and ran a variety of other tests. After about eight hours the doctor emerged and said, "Looks like another anxiety attack. Nothing to worry about, really. We'll keep an eye on it. If it happens again, we'll see about it." Again, he sent us on our way.

I took my niece back to my mother's house and drove home. The whole experience nagged at me. I'm a problem solver. We had a problem. And this was no way to solve it.

I took a step back and called some friends who had been through similar experiences. The consensus was that's generally what you get. If there's no drug to prescribe, and there's nothing to be said in terms of acute care, the doctors say, "Let's see what happens. We'll monitor it." It was cold comfort when one friend said at least I wouldn't get a huge medical bill like I would if I was in the United States.

I thought there must be something more here. And that's when I realized, I hadn't even looked at this from a genetic perspective to try and find the root cause. I was busy dealing with it as a crisis and relying on doctors, as I should have. But I knew from personal experience that a person's genes and the load they put on them—environmental, nutritional, and lifestyle—means everything when it comes to their health and happiness. My own health, in fact my whole life, had changed dramatically because of this insight. I'd even built a business on it. I'd already analyzed my own children's genetics so I could more effectively give them their best chance in life. In that moment I thought, *What can Nur's genetics tell me about her? Would her genetics be sort of an instruction manual that could guide our family in how we raise her? And in an increasingly unpredictable world, could the genetics of children everywhere be an instruction manual for all parents?* If we truly believe children are our best hope for the future, shouldn't we raise them using the best possible information we have available to us? Instead of using them as early-warning systems, can't we give them a guidebook for their lives?

Getting people to think about the role genetics plays in their lives is hard. For one thing, the average person—people who aren't geneticists—can't see genes. The closest they get is when they look at their baby and say, "He's got my eyes" or "She's got your nose." Or perhaps when their child makes a mess and for the umpteenth time does not clean it up after being told to, the mother says, "Those are your father's genes."

For another thing, as of late we've been conditioned to primarily think about genetics in terms of ancestry. That's how millions of people claim descendancy from historical figures such as Charlemagne, William the Conqueror, and Alexander the Great. Or, using my own last name, that's how 1 in every 200 men alive today is a direct descendant of the Mongolian superstud Genghis Khan.

Finally, even if the average person had a special microscope and could see genes, they wouldn't know what they were looking at. Maybe somewhere in the recesses of their memory they'd recall learning about cells and DNA and chromosomes in high school biology and chemistry classes, but they would have no idea what genes do. What's more, even if they saw or heard an explanation of those things, they wouldn't necessarily understand them or how they work together. For instance, you might read that genes are a section of DNA that are in charge of different functions like making proteins. Or that long strands of DNA composed of lots of genes make up chromosomes.

And that chromosomes are located inside the nucleuses of cells. But you wouldn't know in what context they all exist or how and why they do what they do.

In the beginning, it was hard even for me to understand genetics and the role genes play in our lives. That's despite the fact that I run a biotechnology company and work with one of the world's foremost functional genomics scientists, Dr. Mansoor Mohammed. I've also read everything about genetics that I can get my hands on, I constantly go to conferences, and I have even studied genetics at Harvard University.

Despite my background, initially I still didn't think of genetics when my mother called me about my niece. Here was this sweet, innocent 14-year-old girl, collapsed on the floor for no apparent reason. My first reaction was to see a medical doctor. What does a medical doctor do? They check to see if their patient falls into a category of illness so they can check a box and prescribe some sort of medication. If they can't figure it out, they "watch it."

This doesn't exactly promote confidence in parents.

I, as a father of small children, know that being a parent is the hardest job we'll ever love. It starts before we even conceive, continues from the time our children are born to the time they leave the house, and lasts the rest of our lives.

And yet some of us think we've done our jobs if our children are fed and clothed and alive at the end of each day. We give them the basics, rationalize that a little of this or a little of that never hurt us when we were kids, and we hope for the best.

Others among us hover over our children and try to mold them into who we think they should be. We tell them what to think and feel and say and do, we schedule every second of their days with sports and arts and academics and other activities. We even arrange "dates" so they can play and make friends. We don't hope for the best; we demand it.

And then there are those of us who wish we had an instruction manual to tell us what to do—and not do—to give our children the best chance at living a healthy and happy life. Lacking a manual, we try to piece together advice from mothers, mothers-in-law, doulas, nannies, pediatricians, nurses, tutors, coaches, teachers, guidance counselors, therapists, high-priced parenting consultants, and our "intuition."

What are we so concerned about?

A poll conducted by the C. S. Mott Children's Hospital at the University of Michigan revealed that even before the COVID-19 pandemic, parents' top concerns included racism, gun violence, poverty, unequal health care access, child abuse and neglect, overuse of social media, bullying and cyberbullying, Internet safety, unhealthy eating, depression and suicide, lack of physical activity, stress and anxiety, smoking and vaping, and drinking and using drugs.

We are doing no less than raising the future—for our children, for ourselves, and for our planet. Can anyone blame parents for lamenting the fact that there is no instruction manual?

Or *is* there?

It turns out we've had an instructional manual right in front of us—inside our children—all along. It's their DNA—the language of life—and if we learn how to translate that language and understand what it's telling us, we can be the kind of parents we aspire to be.

Every second of every day our children have within them approximately 22,000 genes that tell their more than 30 trillion cells, each with its own structure and function, what to do. By tapping into and harnessing this knowledge, we can keep them physically, mentally, and emotionally healthy. We can help them get the most out of the genetics they've been given. We can set them up for success—aligned with their uniqueness as individuals—at every stage of their lives.

In fact, we influence our children's lives from before they're born until after they've left our house. We do this through a combination of nature and nurture—the genes we pass down to them, and the choices we make about how we eat and exercise, our lifestyle, and how we tend to our own mental, physical, and emotional well-being.

You may be wondering how things turned out with my niece. Well, as I was going over in my mind what might be the root cause of her debilitating anxiety attacks, I asked my mom an uncomfortable but necessary question. What was Nur's menstrual cycle, and when was her last period? She said it started the day before the attack. I then went back into my phone to see when I'd gotten that call from my mom for the first episode. I looked at the dates and I realized it was also right around the time of the start of her menstrual cycle. Could there be a cause and effect here?

When I went back and studied her genetics, I found she is highly androgen dominant as a female, which means she does not produce nearly enough estrogen. So that time right before a female's period, when estrogens are so low, well, it was even lower for her. If you compound her hormone imbalance with the fact that she had to stay inside all day because of COVID-19 and was therefore not getting vitamin D from sunlight, she was physiologically set up to have an anxiety response. This meant that what we were being told was a mental health condition was a vitamin D and hormonal condition.

A couple of months later, while I was still figuring this all out and hadn't had a chance to put a plan in place to help my niece, my mom called and told me that Nur had run away from home. I dropped everything and immediately went over there. Within minutes I found her outside of my mother's building. She hadn't even left the property.

When I talked to her, I could tell she was running away from nothing but herself because she didn't even know what was wrong. She felt horrible in her brain. She felt horrible in her body, but she didn't know what the cause was.

Over the next few days, we dug deep and started to mitigate. Nur agreed that through her problem, we were going to solve everybody else's problem. By itself, this empowered her and gave her a larger sense of purpose.

With oversight from a medical doctor, we started to give her extremely high doses of vitamin D. We started to deal with her dopamine levels. And we started to deal with her hormonal levels. Over the course of several months, she did not have any recurrences of anxiety attacks. If you've ever experienced an anxiety attack you know how much of a relief that was for Nur. Moreover, ongoing chronic stress leads to inflammation in the body, so there is an enormous physical cost. For instance, over time, with too much inflammation, a person with anxiety is at increased risk for diabetes, fatty liver, kidney disease, arthritis, heart disease, and some cancers.

This experience led us to understand that what could very well be categorized as a mental health issue often is not. Especially when it comes to females and hormone issues. This misdiagnosis could partly explain why 25 percent of middle-aged women are taking a medication for mental health that they began taking in their youth.

Fortified with this insight, we made it our mission to ensure that not only are we here to educate but also to give people help and support. Not just about mental health, as I described above, but with all manner of chronic illnesses. We find solutions and give support by understanding the root cause, which is what is happening with a person's genetics, then fix the foundation, not the symptom. This is true health optimization, and it is only available by personalizing through a genetic lens.

Best of all, the canaries are free to fly.

Chapter 2

BIOMEDICAL EXPLORERS

Education is what remains after one has forgotten what one has learned in school.

— ALBERT EINSTEIN, NOBEL PRIZE–WINNING SCIENTIST

Dr. Rosalind Franklin was one of the most influential biomedical explorers in history.

Among the many things I admire about the life and work of Dr. Franklin, the brilliant and trailblazing scientist whose Photo 51 revealed the double-helix structure of DNA, is how she was unwilling to accept the status quo and put limitations on her interests. Without her, we might never have unlocked the secret to how life is passed down from one generation to the next.

To think it almost didn't happen.

I want to specifically call attention to her because she is an example of the kind of attitude we need to adopt if we're going to prevent and reverse disease, age more slowly, and optimize our performance. We don't have to be world-class scientists, but we can take more than a passing interest in science and be active participants in our own health.

Dr. Franklin was born to Anglo-Jewish scholars in London in 1920, and she had to overcome many obstacles to pursue her passion for scientific exploration and discovery. Although she demonstrated an early aptitude for science and was accepted to study physical chemistry at Newnham College, one of two schools for women at Cambridge University, her father did not believe a woman belonged in the sciences and he refused to pay for her education. Undaunted, she asked her aunt for help so she could pay her way, and she got it.

With an indomitable spirit, she persevered through circumstances that would sink a lesser person. During World War II, nothing could stop her from getting the education she desired—bombs, shortages, and family tensions be damned. As Europe was ravaged by the Nazis and her classmates fled Cambridge for safer confines she stayed put, argued world affairs in dispatches to her parents, and worked as an air raid warden to help her country fight the enemy. Through it all, Rosalind Franklin embodied the British saying popularized during World War II, Keep Calm and Carry On.

As a result of her efforts at Cambridge, she earned a Ph.D. in physical chemistry from the university in 1945. Although she was not the first British woman to obtain a doctorate in chemistry—that distinction belongs to Edith Ellen Humphrey at the University of Zurich in 1901—women working as professional scientists in 1945 were few and far between. Thus, her accomplishment was even more impressive.

After moving to King's College in London, she conducted groundbreaking research but again felt unwelcome—women scientists were not allowed to eat lunch in the same room as the men, and the women were expected to play subservient roles in the "man's world." The combination of anti-Semitism and sexism proved to be a factor in the lack of credit she was given for her work.

Working in a laboratory environment less than collegial to female scientists and often in isolation, Dr. Franklin patiently struggled to prove the structure through mathematical computations and to capture the B form of DNA through more than 100 hours of photographic exposure. While her Photo 51 and related data were integral to the 1953 discovery and description of the double-helix structure of DNA, her contribution went largely unrecognized for nearly 50 years.

The story of Dr. Franklin, who, despite gender disparity and discrimination, relentlessly pursued the answers to questions that have improved health and longevity around the world, speaks to new generations who take up the struggle for equality and improved well-being. Her perseverance and determination in the face of entrenched injustice should offer hope to all of those who want to live healthier, longer, and more productive lives.

The discovery of the structure of DNA sparked a revolution in the biological sciences and technology and expanded knowledge in many other fields. Based on the structure of DNA, the new science of molecular biology was born, and led to prevention, diagnosis, and treatment in ways that were unimaginable in 1952. The advances in identification and analysis of the genetic code based on Dr. Franklin's work have produced breakthroughs that changed the trajectory of science and will continue to improve the human condition.

When I undertook my remedial science studies—rediscovering Gregor Mendel and learning about Rosalind Franklin and others—I began to wonder about the quality of the science education I received as a youngster. Doing that made me consider how young people are being taught science today. I thought, if people want to prevent and reverse disease, age more slowly, and optimize their performance, they need to take control of their own health instead of outsourcing it solely to the medical establishment. And to do that, it would be a big help if they had basic knowledge of biology, chemistry, and physics.

As I examined how today's students are being taught science, I found something that might explain why they forget so much of what they've been taught—while they may *like* science, they don't like science *class*. Why is that?

A report by the Amgen Foundation and Change the Equation, both of which advocate for stronger education in science, technology, engineering, and math (STEM), offers an explanation. The results were based on an online survey of more than 1,500 teenage students from around the United States.

Some 81 percent of teens said they were interested in science and 73 percent said they wanted to learn more about biology. But only 37 percent of students said they enjoy their science class, and even fewer—33 percent—liked biology class. That's less than the 48 percent who said they enjoyed non-science classes. That's not a great number either. But it's better than science class.

One key factor is that while many teens find more hands-on experiences like field trips and experiments to be most compelling, most instruction in science class involves either textbooks or in-class discussion. To me, memorizing facts from a textbook or a teacher's lecture is antithetical to learning. Think of the teacher from the film *Ferris Bueller's Day Off* droning "Bueller, anyone, Bueller" on and on at the front of the class. It's enough to make *any* subject boring.

The survey also examined the relationship between students' family income and access to and interest in STEM fields. Lower-income students, like I was when I was a young student, were less likely to know an adult involved in biology and less likely to participate in a science club.

Overall, more than 80 percent of teens reported that they thought knowing adults in their desired field of work might help them advance, but only about a third knew adults in that field.

The authors of the Amgen and Change the Equation report argue that schools should adopt more inquiry-based STEM curricula and that teachers should receive training in how to teach it. They also argue for stronger ties between businesses and community member schools.

As I see it, given our achievement-oriented culture, too many teachers are forced to "teach to the test" so they and their schools get higher ratings. Or, at the very least, so their school does not receive poor ratings. Higher-rated schools means higher-priced real estate. That's fine for housing prices and a town's desirability, but not helpful when it comes to students being able to learn and apply knowledge to real-world problems.

Moreover, stronger ties between businesses and community member schools is a good idea if it means students receive more practical education. But if those ties are designed to simply funnel students into careers instead of inspiring them to pursue learning so they can apply it to their lives, it's not as valuable. Think how useful it would be if every student understood their own genetics, and how their environmental, nutritional, and lifestyle choices interact with those genetics. Learning something would no longer be for a test or a job, but for a life.

That's why learning science is so important. Each one of us, and our children, are the laboratory, subject, experiment, and outcome rolled into one.

This is what today's biomedical explorers, aka "biohackers," are doing—constantly optimizing their health and the way their brains and bodies function. In addition to reading this book and engaging with us at The DNA Company, I encourage everyone to follow some of the people who are influencing my personal development. The following are some of the best-known.

Dave Asprey, four-time *New York Times* best-selling author, creator of Bulletproof Coffee, founder of Bulletproof 360, and host of the Webby–award winning podcast *Bulletproof Radio*. A pioneer in the biohacking movement, Dave has devoted his life and resources to elevating human performance using the latest scientific research combined with ancient healing traditions. By biomedically exploring how he could hack his own brain and body for peak performance, he's lost more than 100 pounds, gotten biologically younger, and raised his IQ. Now, his mission is to share the latest discoveries in health and wellness to help people break through mental and physical barriers to accomplish the unimaginable—to be superhuman. Dave is an advisor to my company.

Tim Ferriss, entrepreneur, author of five *New York Times* bestselling books, technology investor and advisor, and host of *The Tim Ferriss Podcast*—the first business interview podcast to exceed 100 million downloads, now at 800 million. A master of deconstructing skills and information so they can be easily understood and applied, Tim broke into biohacking with his book *The Four-Hour Body*. In the book and on his podcast, Tim and his guests dive deep into health, biohacking, lifestyle design, and mental performance.

Ben Greenfield, a human body and brain performance coach, ex-bodybuilder, 13-time Ironman triathlete, professional Spartan athlete, anti-aging consultant, speaker, and *New York Times* best-selling author of 17 books, including *Beyond Training, Boundless,* and *Fit Soul*. His podcast, *Ben Greenfield Life*, is a trusted source of information that provides listeners with an outside-the-box approach to discovering health, happiness, and hope—all with a holistic approach that blends the body, the mind, and the spirit while bringing about lasting results and fulfillment so that they can live their best, most impactful life. As a biomedical explorer, it's no wonder Ben was voted by the National Strength and Conditioning Association to be America's Top Personal Trainer, and selected by Greatist as one of the top 100 Most Influential People in Health and Fitness.

Dr. B. J. Fogg is a behavior scientist, Stanford University professor, and author of the *New York Times* best-selling book *Tiny Habits*. At Stanford University he has directed a research lab for more than 20 years. On the industry side, he trains innovators to use his work so they can create solutions that influence behavior for good. His focus areas include health, sustainability, financial well-being, learning, productivity, and more. Although Dr. Fogg might not call himself a biohacker or biomedical explorer, he deeply understands that it's not enough even to know your DNA and how your lifestyle, environment, and nutrition impact your health, you have to change your behavior. I'm proud to say he has brought his knowledge and expertise to The DNA Company to guide us in helping our clients achieve lasting change.

Dr. Mark Hyman is leading a health revolution—one revolving around using food as medicine to support longevity, energy, mental clarity, happiness, and so much more. He is a practicing family physician and an internationally recognized leader, speaker, educator, founder and director of The UltraWellness Center, the head of strategy and innovation at the Cleveland Clinic Center for Functional Medicine, a 14-time *New York Times* best-selling author, and board president for clinical affairs at the Institute for Functional Medicine. He is the host of one of the leading health podcasts, *The Doctor's Farmacy*.

Finally, Ray Kurzweil is one of the world's leading inventors, thinkers, and futurists, with a 30-year track record of accurate predictions. A graduate of the world-renowned Massachusetts Institute of Technology, he has written five successful books, including *New York Times* bestsellers *The Singularity Is Near* and *How to Create a Mind*.

He is also co-founder and chancellor of Singularity University, and a director of engineering at Google heading up a team developing machine intelligence and natural language understanding.

Called "the restless genius" by *The Wall Street Journal* and "the ultimate thinking machine" by *Forbes* magazine, he was selected as one of the top entrepreneurs by *Inc.* magazine, which described him as the "rightful heir to Thomas Edison." *PBS* selected him as one of the "sixteen revolutionaries who made America."

Given what I've just written about Ray Kurzweil, and what is publicly known about his interest in studying and modeling technology trends and their impact on society, you may be wondering what he is doing in a chapter about biomedical exploration. It turns out he is a champion biohacker as well!

Much like I did, and like many people, Kurzweil didn't pay much attention to his health until his mid-30s. After his father died of an early heart attack, Kurzweil began looking into his own health and discovered he had an early form of type 2 diabetes, a major risk factor for heart disease. He then hooked up with Dr. Terry Grossman, who was willing to take an unconventional approach to helping Kurzweil become healthier. This included—among many alternative methods—Kurzweil taking hundreds of specially designed supplements, undergoing chemical intravenous treatments, and drinking red wine, green tea, and alkaline water to reverse his illness, live longer, and put more vitality in his life. Together, Kurzweil and Grossman have authored two books—*Fantastic Voyage: Live Long Enough to Live Forever* and *Transcend: Nine Steps to Living Well Forever.*

I came upon this knowledge in 2017 when I was doing research regarding my own health issues and discovered Kurzweil was behind something called "The DEF CON Biohacking Village," a multiday biotechnology conference focused on breakthrough do-it-yourself, grinder, transhumanist, medical technology, and information security solutions. At the conference, they talked about how, by 2017, there had been multiple instances of do-it-yourself biohacking overcoming conventional science and how in the future the progress would accelerate. With a true open-source approach, the event organizers celebrated the biohacker movement with a wide variety of talks, demonstrations, and a medical device hackathon.

Their theme—Medical Industry Disruption—was music to my ears. As Kurzweil and his colleagues said, the medical industry is one of the last to be touched by technology. In Western society, doctors have been put on pedestals, and the study of medicine has traditionally taken place in medical institutions and university labs. They were advocating using citizen science—another way of saying biomedical exploration or biohacking—to solve the economic problems that are caused by privatizing medicine and the resources for research—such as the more than $4 trillion we spend on health care while achieving diminishing returns.

I remember reading the following from their manifesto and feeling like pure energy had been shot into my veins: "We welcome anyone interested in do-it-yourself biology. Biohackers reject the idea that all medical, biological, and genetic advancements must come from a large institution, university, or corporation. We reject the idea that modifications to biology must only be in response to disease or dysfunction. We reject the natural order given to us by evolution . . . or perhaps we have evolved to the point where we can take evolution into our own hands. We dare to ask the questions: How can we use technology to enhance our raw abilities, specific skills, overall health, or well-being? How can we usher in an age where we not only fix what's broken, but we make ourselves, and our world, better?"

We don't have to be as brilliant or accomplished as any of the people I've cited; most of us aren't. But we can take some control over our health by being curious about our bodies and the science that underpins everything we do and all that we are. This pursuit of knowledge doesn't have to take place in an ivory tower; it can take place in your basement. And it is also appropriate—in fact needed—by people of any age, gender, ethnicity, or socioeconomic status. If you're a parent, embark on your learning journey now, but also encourage your kids to do the same. If you're middle-aged and the process of becoming increasingly ill has already begun, you have plenty of time to reverse it. If you're a senior citizen and many of the health challenges have already hit you, it is never too late to reverse decades of damage and significantly extend the length and vitality of your life.

Set sail, biomedical explorers!

Chapter 3

• •°• •.•°•.•°•°•.•°•.°

DOCTOR YOU

*When we understand the connection between
how we live and how long we live, it's easier
to make different choices.*

— DEAN ORNISH, M.D., FOUNDER AND PRESIDENT OF THE
PREVENTIVE MEDICINE RESEARCH INSTITUTE AND AUTHOR OF
FOUR *NEW YORK TIMES* BEST-SELLING BOOKS

Billions of dollars have been spent decoding our genome with the promise of understanding disease and instituting an era of precision medicine. Let me tell you why that's so important.

Precision medicine is health care tailored to you. It's not designed to enrich big pharmaceutical companies, physicians, health insurance providers, and other members of the health care–industrial complex. It's a partnership with your doctors and clinicians, with you at the center, having the final say in your health care.

We're not there yet, but we're getting closer every day.

In his 2015 State of the Union address, President Obama announced that he was investing an initial $215 million to launch the Precision Medicine Initiative—a bold new research effort to revolutionize how we improve health and treat disease. Just as with many government programs, the promise of executing such an initiative is dependent on politics. Everyone knows who followed President Obama in the White House, so you'll have to guess what happened; I hope it somehow miraculously survived. But I can say with certainty that President Obama did a superb job of stating where we are with precision medicine and where we need to go.

As President Obama noted, and as I indicated earlier, medical treatments have primarily and historically been designed for the "average patient." As a result of this "one size fits all" approach, treatments can be successful for some patients but not for others. Precision medicine, on the other hand, is an innovative approach that considers individual differences in people's genes, environments, nutrition, and lifestyles. It gives medical professionals the resources they need to target the specific treatments of the illnesses we encounter, further develops our scientific and medical research, and prevents and reverses disease, slows the aging process, and adds more vitality to your life.

President Obama stated that advances in precision medicine have already led to powerful new discoveries and several new treatments that are tailored to specific characteristics, such as a person's genetic makeup or the genetic profile of an individual's tumor. This is true, and it is helping to transform the way we treat diseases such as cancer. Patients with breast, lung, and colorectal cancers, as well as melanomas and leukemias, for instance, routinely undergo molecular testing as part of patient care, enabling physicians to select treatments that improve chances of survival and reduce occurrence of adverse effects.

The future of precision medicine will enable health care providers to tailor treatment and prevention strategies to people's unique characteristics, including their genome sequence, microbiome composition, health history, environment, lifestyle, and diet. To get there, we need to incorporate many different types of data, including a person's metabolomics (the chemicals in the body at a certain point in time), their microbiome (the collection of microorganisms in or on the body), and information about the patient collected by health care providers and the patients themselves. Success will require that health data be portable and easily shared between providers, researchers, and, most important, patients and research participants.

Note that I said "share" data, not "sell" data. Unlike some DNA testing companies, we never sell our clients' data.

Precision medicine will pioneer a new model of patient-powered research that promises to accelerate biomedical discoveries and provide clinicians with new tools and knowledge to use in selecting the new therapies that will work best for particular patients.

The potential for precision medicine to improve care and speed the development of new treatments has only just begun to be tapped. Translating initial successes to a larger scale will require a coordinated and sustained international effort. Through collaborative public and private efforts, precision medicine will leverage advances in genomics, emerging methods for managing and analyzing large data sets while protecting privacy, and health information technology to accelerate biomedical discoveries. President Obama's Precision Medicine Initiative, if adequately implemented and funded, also promised to engage a million or more Americans to volunteer to contribute their health data to improve health outcomes, fuel the development of new treatments, and catalyze a new era of data-based and more precise medical treatment.

While precision medicine is indeed something we should strive for, and I completely support President Obama's initiative, what can you do *right now* to improve your health?

In a study by the Harvard T. H. Chan School of Public Health, researchers found five practices every woman can do immediately to extend her life by 14 years. These same practices will extend men's lives by 12 years. That's at least 12 to 14 more vibrant years of traveling, reading great books and writing them, painting, going to museums and art galleries, playing music or going to concerts, singing, dancing, gardening, belonging to a bridge club, seeing films, hiking, biking, swimming, playing golf and tennis, eating at fabulous restaurants, volunteering, worshipping, being with your loved ones, and anything else your *healthy* heart desires.

The Harvard Chan study, published in *Circulation* in 2018, was the first broad-reaching examination of the effect of embracing a low-risk lifestyle—by adopting five healthy practices—on longevity in the United States. While the study looked at Americans, we can consider the United States to be a stand-in for any Western society.

On average, Americans can expect to have shorter lives—79.3 years—than almost all other comparable countries. The U.S. ranked

31st in the world for life expectancy in 2015. The goal of the Harvard Chan study was to quantify how much healthy lifestyle practices might be able to increase longevity in the U.S.

Harvard Chan researchers and colleagues examined 34 years of data from 78,865 women and 27 years of data from 44,354 men participating in, respectively, the Nurses' Health Study and the Health Professionals Follow-Up Study.

Are you ready for this groundbreaking scientific discovery? This magic elixir? The fountain of youth that not even Ponce de León could find?

Here are the five practices: eating a healthy diet, exercising regularly, keeping a healthy body weight, not drinking too much alcohol, and not smoking.

That's it.

We are so sick as a society that this is how low the bar is set to add 12 to 14 years to your life. Not because these five practices are powerful catalysts of change, but because *we* are. Or we *can* be because none of these five things will work unless we *do* them. As Shakespeare wrote, "Ay, there's the rub."

The study yielded some stark contrasts between those who did adopt the low-risk lifestyle factors and those who didn't. For instance, researchers predicted that by age 50, women participants who didn't practice the low-risk lifestyle factors would live only 29 more years, and men, 25.5 more years. You may say 79 and 75.5 years old; not bad, right? Sure, but researchers also predicted that 50-year-old women participants who incorporated all five low-risk factors into their lives would live to be 93.1 years old. And men, 87.6 years old. A 14-year gap and 12-year gap is quite a difference.

In addition, compared with those who didn't follow any of the healthy lifestyle habits, those who followed all five were 74 percent less likely to die during the study period. What's more, the researchers also found that people who practiced all five healthy behaviors at the same time had the best chance of extending their lives.

"This study underscores the importance of following healthy lifestyle habits for improving longevity in the U.S. population," said Dr. Frank Hu, senior author of the study and Fredrick J. Stare Professor of Nutrition and Epidemiology at the Harvard Chan school. "However, adherence to healthy lifestyle habits is very low. Therefore, public policies should put more emphasis on creating healthy food, built, and social environments to support and promote healthy diet and lifestyles."

In a follow-up and extension of the study in 2020, Harvard Chan researchers found that middle-aged people who practice the five healthy habits may increase the years they live free of type 2 diabetes, cardiovascular disease, and cancer. In other words, they're not just adding years to their life, they're adding life to their years. In the study, women practicing four or five healthy habits at age 50 lived an average of 34.4 more years free of diabetes, cardiovascular diseases, and cancer, compared to 23.7 healthy years among women who practiced none. Men practicing four or five healthy habits at age 50 lived 31.1 years free of chronic disease, compared to 23.5 years among men who practiced none. Men who were current heavy smokers and obese men and women had the lowest disease-free life expectancy.

"Given the high cost of chronic disease treatment, public policies to promote a healthy lifestyle by improving food and physical environments would help to reduce health care costs and improve quality of life," concluded Hu.

It's important to understand that Dr. Hu cited the need for public policies twice, in 2018 and 2020.

In my own research, I was surprised to learn that these revelations built upon studies done decades earlier.

Consider Dr. Dean Ornish, who earned his medical degree from the Baylor College of Medicine, completed a medical internship and residency at Massachusetts General Hospital (1981–1984), and was a clinical fellow in medicine at Harvard Medical School.

Now founder and president of the Preventive Medicine Research Institute in Sausalito, California, clinical professor of medicine at the University of California, San Francisco, and author of four *New York Times* best-selling books, Ornish is known for his lifestyle-driven approach to the control and reversal of coronary heart disease and other chronic diseases. Through his scientifically proven Lifestyle Medicine program, he promotes lifestyle changes such as eating primarily (but not exclusively) a whole-foods, plant-based diet; stopping smoking; moderately exercising; managing stress through yoga, meditation, and other methods; limiting alcohol intake; and implementing these lifestyle changes within a loving, supportive community. Aside from the last bit about psychosocial support, his recommendations are the same as the five healthy lifestyle practices Harvard researchers advocated decades later.

Talk about being ahead of your time!

From the 1970s through the 1990s, Ornish and others researched the impact of diet and stress levels on people with heart disease. The research, published in peer-reviewed journals, became the basis of his Program for Reversing Heart Disease. It combined diet, meditation, and exercise and support groups, and in 1993, a full 25 years before the *new* Harvard Chan study, it became the first nonsurgical, nonpharmaceutical therapy for heart disease to qualify for insurance reimbursement. With the exception of chiropractic care, it was the first alternative medical technique not taught in traditional medical-school curricula to gain approval by a major insurance carrier.

Dr. Ornish is a prime example of a biomedical explorer. Think of how many people could have lived longer and lived better doing so if they'd followed his recommendations. I'm sure many have, but certainly not at the scale we need it to be. You can chalk some of that up to the normal resistance people have to change. But I'd also venture to say that people have not had available to them the insights that can be had from functional genomics, largely because they were still being discovered. But now, those discoveries are accelerating exponentially, and soon, getting your DNA tested will be as commonplace as any other medical procedure.

With proper public policies and education, people will begin to understand that they aren't born with type 2 diabetes or heart disease. For the most part they are born healthy. Which begs the question: Why not just stay healthy and grow old healthy, and eventually die from a coconut falling on your head while on a trip to Aruba?

Well, what happens is that over time we make environment, nutrition, and lifestyle choices that are mismatched to our genetic legacy, and we start to expose our cells to a load with which they were never designed to cope. We become metabolically unhealthy and riddled with inflammation, the root cause of disease.

As I said earlier, those environment, nutrition, and lifestyle choices are not the same for all of us. The one-size-fits-all, trial-and-error approach to health is no different than playing Russian roulette. It works for some, but it's deadly for others.

And the belief that masking symptoms is health care success is a farce. Pain is not the problem. Pain is your body screaming out that there is something wrong that needed to be addressed long before the pain arrived. Our symptom-masking approach to health is akin to keeping a pet fish in a bowl of toxic, polluted water; the fish starts to get eczema, migraines, maybe even cancer, but you treat each problem with a separate pill while leaving the fish in the toxic water. It's an improvement over what we did to the poor canaries, but not by much. This is what we do to ourselves.

To achieve the optimal version of yourself, you don't need to look outward for the next fad book or viral video. When you were born you came with an instruction manual. It's inside every cell in your body, and if you read and interpret it, you will know exactly what you need to do.

Whether it's your mental health, preventing or reversing disease, slowing down aging, determining what diet you should be on, figuring out why you can't sleep at night, getting rid of your anxiety, or even understanding the neurochemicals of your brain and knowing whether you should be an accountant or an entrepreneur, all you need to do is look inside. That's where you will find the answers. By making choices that are aligned to your unique genetic makeup, you will prevent and reverse disease, slow aging, and optimize performance.

This is just the beginning; we are capable of so much more.

Informed Choice

Your genetics are a phenomenal thing.

A 40-year-old person who looks and feels like they're 28 hasn't gotten that way because they left things to chance. They're doing things differently. The opposite is also true. A 28-year-old person who looks like they're 40 has gotten that way not by accident, but by choice.

Chronic disease. Biological aging. Poor performance. These are all the results of wrong choices. Choices that hurt or hinder you, rather than heal or help you. But how do you know what the right choices are for you? What would be the impact if you always made the right choice?

What if you could change the day you die?

When you see those first wrinkles, or those gray hairs, or you get the call from a doctor who says, "I need to see you; your test results are in," you take it for granted that this is all meant to happen. That aging and chronic disease are just a part of life.

Well, what if they're not?

You can't feel cancer coming. There's no warning that dementia is on the way. So we think these things just happen. We get sick, we try to treat it, but it's too late. Well, now there's a better way. A way that puts us each in charge of our own destiny.

Genetic research has advanced more in the last 3 years than in the last 30. And this personalized instruction manual that's in each one of us has finally been properly decoded. Using it, we can now get ahead of disease or even reverse it, decide how we age, and have a direct impact on whether we thrive or languish in our performance.

Our scientists at The DNA Company have clinically studied more than 7,000 people. We've sat in front of every one of them. We've looked at their hair, their skin, their mood and behavior, their medical history—everything about them—all overlaid on their DNA map. We've understood where the biochemistry of their trillions of cells intersects with the instructions of their 22,000 genes. And because of that, we know the choices each person needs to make to slow down aging and catch disease before it even happens.

I have no doubt that with the genetic insights we're seeing today, chronic disease will soon be a story that we tell our grandchildren. Because if you understand why chronic disease, aging, and poor performance really happen, you also understand that they are truly optional.

It all starts with understanding what we call your hardware. What are you made of? What are your systems? Where are they optimal? Where are they suboptimal? It sounds daunting, but this can all be mapped out genetically.

Imagine understanding the quality of your arteries and how prone they are to inflammation, which means how prone they are to disease. Imagine understanding the quality of the vasculature of your brain and how prone you are to stroke and dementia. Imagine understanding the quality of your blood vessels and their ability to dilate and regulate blood pressure or hypertension, the sheer force of blood flow. All these things and more are determinable at the genetic level.

If you have these things mapped out, that's where you can start to understand the root cause of disease. You can prevent and reverse it.

For example, by the age of 38, one of my dear friends had a severe cholesterol issue that wouldn't go away despite implementing the traditional, "tried-and-true" methods of treatment. It was called cholesterolemia and it made no sense, so we looked at his genetics.

We found that there's a gene that determines the quality of your endothelial lining. By *endothelial lining*, I mean the inner lining of the blood vessels and arteries, through which your blood flows and touches the cell membrane. There are different versions. One is robust, like stainless steel. Another is paper thin, so it's more prone to inflammation.

In the paper-thin version, there must be an inflammatory insult to trigger the inflammation. You could have that same vasculature and live on a beach in Aruba and never get sick. But what if you don't live on a beach in Aruba? What if you're in New York breathing air pollution? What if, like my friend, you golf four days a week, thinking you're doing something healthy that you enjoy, but you're breathing in heavy pesticides from the chemicals in the grass that make the golf course so gorgeous? What does that exposure do to you? Well, how your body reacts depends on your genetic capacity to deal with that exposure.

It turns out a single gene is responsible for the clearance of toxins from the blood. What if you have a weak version of that gene? Is that stuff you're breathing wreaking havoc? Where is it wreaking havoc? Exactly which cells are weak? In his case, it was in the vasculature of his arteries. With too much toxicity causing inflammation in his endothelial lining, his body deployed the hormone cholesterol to reduce the inflammation. That's why cholesterol gets built up and sent; it was a natural response. But what happens to cholesterol when it meets toxicity? It gets deposited and hardens. So that high-density lipoprotein (HDL) process where cholesterol is supposed to be transported and cleared through the liver doesn't work. It doesn't move; it stays there because it hardens with the toxicity.

Imagine if my friend had understood his hardware, and his risks, and what his innate capacity was for the different systems and biochemistry of his body, and what load he was capable of handling. That's where, using his genetics, he could plot a course for his wellness journey. Think back. If he'd had this information as a child, he could have known exactly what to do with his environment, nutrition, and lifestyle, so that for the rest of his life he could stay as healthy as when he was born. He could have prevented the serious disease of cholesterolemia.

Once we tested him and figured out the root cause of his illness, we were able to design a protocol of nutritional and environmental changes that enabled him to continue playing the sport he loved, but not quite as much. Instead of four times a week, he played less often. He played on courses that weren't so heavily treated with chemicals. He played at different times, when the chemicals were not so strong. He took up other sports that did not expose him to those chemicals. And he took supplements and changed his diet so he could better fight the chemicals that were so toxic to his system. As a result, his cholesterolemia problem went away.

So that's one example of how disease can be prevented and/or reversed.

What about slowing the aging process? Can your choices make a difference in how quickly you age? You bet they can. You don't wake up one day with wrinkles, gray hair, and no energy; it happens as a process over time.

If it had been possible to get your DNA tested when you were a child, and if you had understood how your biological systems would respond to the lifestyle, nutritional, and environmental loads you'd put on them over the next 50 to 60 years, you could have made choices that would add more years to your life and life to your years. But you couldn't have done any of that because the tests and insights have only become available in the past few years. What you had to do instead was follow the "blunt instrument" advice from the medical establishment to "eat a balanced diet and get some exercise." Unfortunately, that advice didn't say what *kind* of diet you should have or what *type* of exercise program you should be on. As a result, in some cases that advice might have helped you, but in other cases, it didn't, and it may even have hurt you.

What I've just described, in a nutshell, is the health care journey we've been on—from generalized disease-based medicine to personalized functional medicine. We're not where we need to be yet, but we're getting there, and the possibilities are amazing.

For instance, no matter how long you've been making choices that are unhelpful, if you follow some DNA-based anti-aging strategies now, in 10 years' time, you're going to look better and feel better than if you don't.

A lot of it comes down to the reality that the aging of every organ system—skin, hair, heart, skeletal, etc.—comes down to cellular dysfunction and oxidation. And those systems don't work in a vacuum; they're interconnected, and because of that, almost everybody has more than one health issue with which they're dealing. It's kind of a ripple effect. Take osteoarthritis, which impacts a lot of people as they age. If you have osteoarthritis, your risk of dementia is about fivefold higher. Why is that? You have arthritis in your ankles and knees and hips—that's because you ran 10 miles every day, right? Not necessarily. We see plenty of people who run a lot more than that and they're fine. So, what's the answer?

What we do is go back and look at what is wrong in the cell. What happens is the cells of your body all take in oxygen and nutrition to create energy. And in the process of converting oxygen into energy you create an oxidant—a free radical—which is highly toxic. The irony is the oxygen that gives you life is the thing that's aging you.

A gene called SOD2 determines how well you clear the oxidation from the cell. This clearing, or clogging if your gene is suboptimal, happens in the mitochondria, which is what gives the cell energy. And as we start getting damage to our mitochondria with diet and lifestyle and environment and genetics, we start getting senescent cells, also known as "zombie cells," that produce toxins and make all the cells around them sick.

It's like a zombie apocalypse: good for a movie, not good for sustaining life.

Another way to look at it is if you think of the cell as a fireplace. Imagine that fireplace has no chimney, but it is constantly burning wood, and the smoke is getting thicker and thicker because it has no place to go. What's going to happen? The fireplace (the cell) is going to suffocate in oxidation, which will age it and lead to inflammation—the root cause of disease.

We see this dynamic played out in many long-distance runners who come to our company looking for a solution. Some of them may seem fit and have no fat on them, but most of them look kind of haggard with wrinkled and leathery skin and white hair. They wonder why, if they're doing something so healthy, they look like death warmed over. The answer is oxidative stress is leading to more oxidation and rapid aging. Once we've tested them and understood the source of their problem, we can counteract it. We can support their mitochondrial health by helping them clean out the bad zombie cells, having them periodically fast, adding the right foods and supplements to their diet, recommending antioxidative activity, reducing the load they're putting on their cells, and helping them develop habits that work with their genome instead of against it.

Let's look at optimizing your performance, which you could say is the flip side of disease and aging. Perhaps you're an elite athlete, performing artist, Special Forces soldier, honors student, or high-powered executive. Understanding your genetics can help you fine-tune your performance, break through barriers in learning, training, and competition, and quickly fix problems should they occur.

Americans put a premium on high performance—from academics to technology and everything in between. But let's look more closely at athletic performance. It's so important in America that many school districts emphasize athletics far more than academics. Part of that is because the competitiveness and the drive and the true American spirit is manifested through sports and athleticism. But athletics also plays an important role in childhood development—physically, socially, emotionally, cognitively.

Today, by understanding genetics and hormones, we can predict at an early age if someone is designed to be a football player who can lift and push heavy things, or if they are meant to do something like gymnastics or running and be lean and fit. It comes down to hormones. One person has hormones that enable him to be the big, burly guy that can squat a lot of weight and be a great football player who's like a refrigerator that's hard to push. Another may have hormones that enable him to run forever and be a great soccer midfielder who never seems to get tired. One is not better than the other, they're just different.

Parents and coaches may think the big, strong guy is a manly man with a lot of testosterone, but that's not the case. It's estrogen that creates the mass and size and strength. Now, imagine understanding how a child is going to develop based on their hormone profile, which you can now know because when you start your children in sports, you start them early. You don't really know what they're going to look like in their teens because the hormones really don't kick in until that time at a high level. Without knowing any better, you might set your child down the wrong path. And if they're on the wrong path, think of the consequence of years and years of training, time spent driving from city to city to tournaments, only to find out that they're maturing into a completely different person than the role you carved out for them. So, to be able to personalize and understand where they fit in athletics will help them excel as they age into their late teens and early adulthood. And the dream of someone becoming a professional athlete or going to the Olympics is probably more realistic if you're able to personalize insights early.

Then there's the gymnast who is ripped, with every muscle fiber showing. This guy might be able to bench press 300 pounds, but he's got six-pack abs and chiseled shoulders and arms. He's strong, but he may not get the mass from estrogen because instead he's converting his testosterone into DHT, which is highly toxic, and later in life could lead to things like prostate enlargement or hair loss.

The other end of it is the young man or woman who is tall and thin and has a cleaner and purer androgen, a sex hormone of which testosterone is one type. You have to know what kind of hormones people produce. Which hormone leads to what body type, which then points to what someone may be good at or where they fit athletically.

Then there's the issue of how well they clear those hormones. Meaning, now that you understand your child is, for instance, estrogen dominant or testosterone dominant, and whether they produce DHT or not, do you know how well they clear those hormones? Simply producing hormones doesn't mean they'll have access to those hormones for any length of time. For example, men have testosterone cycling in their blood every day, but women cycle through it every month. And, as women get into their teenage years, in puberty, their hormone levels are different throughout the month. That should impact the way they train and the way they recover. The fact is, they're going to have more strength, and better recovery, at certain times of the month. It's important to map that circadian rhythm and understand genetically where these women are so they can plan their training more efficiently and not have these challenges that people so often misunderstand.

We dealt with a young lady who was working toward becoming an Olympic triathlete. A high-performance institute that dealt with professional athletes sent her to us because, they said, they didn't understand why she trained just like everyone else but didn't get the same ripped strength and muscle. They were concerned she didn't look and perform like the other athletes. By analyzing her genetics, we were able to prove that she was unlike the other athletes who were androgen dominant with ripped muscle. While she had the desire and worked extremely hard, she didn't have the same hormone profile to deliver what was being asked of her. She was pushing herself toward something for which she was not designed. Having said that, we adjusted her supplement protocol to augment her genetic expression and get her closer to where she needed to be. She eventually became a champion triathlete.

Her story is an example of the advantage or challenge a certain hormone profile will provide.

In another case, we worked with a hockey player who was trying to get into the National Hockey League. He was extremely motivated and trained very hard, but he couldn't recover. On days after big workouts, he was sore and tired, needed to take naps, and had a difficult time mustering the energy to get back on the ice. When we looked at his genetics, we found that he was unable to clear the toxins that were being produced during heavy cardiovascular activity. And he had a bigger challenge; not only was his detox profile suboptimal, so was his anti-inflammatory profile. The harder he trained, the worse he got. That's counterintuitive to an elite athlete. So we gave him a specially designed supplement to boost his muscle capability and his detox capability. Problem solved.

Now, if you do have weak detox at the mitochondrial level, as our NHL player does, as the cells in your body take in nutrition and oxygen to create energy, they also create oxidation or oxidative stress. It all works together—by knowing this you can prevent or reverse disease, slow aging, and optimize your performance.

Here's an example of how it all works together. You know how you sometimes hear of 35-year-old soccer players or 35-year-old Olympic sprinters who drop dead of heart attacks? They're in the best condition, have the best training, the best foods, the best doctors in the world. Why would they have heart attacks? It's because nobody checked on their detox profile, and they were doing aggressive cardiovascular training while being unable to clear the oxidative stress or that oxidant. When that happens, they might be minus 70 percent capacity for that function of clearing. Over time the oxidant builds up like soot in a fireplace. This puts a tremendous load on their cells as they age and makes them more prone to inflammation, which is a root cause of disease. If they understood their genetics, they would know whether doing heavy cardiovascular training was good for them or poisonous. For some people, heavy cardiovascular training is a way to become ill, increasing rapid aging and damage to their cells, which leads to inflammation and disease, and poor performance. With genetic testing and the right protocols, they can do the exact opposite.

The possibilities for what can be achieved are remarkable. As I've outlined, your body is not just a collection of individual cells and genes but a complex network of interconnected systems that all work together. We will take a close look at each of those systems in the coming chapters.

Part Two

THE
SOLUTION

Chapter 4

DNA, MOOD, AND BEHAVIOR

We are not victims, but we are actually masters of our genetic activity.

— DR. BRUCE LIPTON, PH.D., DEVELOPMENTAL BIOLOGIST
AND AUTHOR OF *THE BIOLOGY OF BELIEF*

Before I got my DNA tested and began to get well, if I was irritable or felt depressed, I made jokes about it. I'd say I must have "gotten up on the wrong side of the bed" or my "wires were crossed." That's because I didn't understand what was going on with me, and I wanted to minimize the fact that I was snapping at people or moping around. Of course, sometimes circumstances did influence the way I acted or felt, but I didn't have any idea how or why. It was as if I was a puppet and someone else was controlling my strings.

In a sense, that is what was happening. Our mood, behavior, and personality are influenced by many factors, including diet, lifestyle, environment, family history, personal history, and genetics. At the biological level, our minds uniquely express emotions, memories, thoughts, and feelings depending on the important relationship between the neurochemicals our bodies produce, such as dopamine, serotonin, and brain-derived neurotrophic factor, and the cells in our brain, known as neurons.

The genes in our DNA play an influential role in how these neurochemicals interact with our brains and ultimately influence our overall mood and behavior. It is important to note, however, that the genes' influence is not diagnostic but associative. In other words, while these genes may indicate a predisposition toward certain behaviors, the reality is that factors like diet, lifestyle, family history, personal history, and the environment can and will interact to dampen or augment the influence of these genes on our overall mood and behavior.

Before we can make meaningful lifestyle and wellness recommendations, we must first assess our unique ability to process emotional stimuli—which means getting our DNA tested. We start by looking at the prefrontal cortex, which is the seat of the brain's executive functions. It is also a center for the neuronal activity involved in mood, behavior, abstract thinking, and working memory.

By testing and evaluating variants within the COMT, DRD2, ADRA2B, 5-HTTLPR, MAO, TPH2, and BDNF genes we can see how different individuals respond to pleasure, form emotional imprints, and exhibit differences in executive functions. The implications are far-reaching and impact your work and career, your diet, how you sleep, your addictive and depressive and bingeing tendencies, your propensity for anxiety and burnout, your risk of ADHD, your ability to focus, and more.

When I got my own DNA tested, the insights changed my life. I can't tell you how your life would be changed because I don't know your DNA and the choices you make. Probably the best way for me to give you an idea of how these insights might manifest for you is to share the results and summaries of my own genetic tests.

First, my results.

Gene Tested	COMT	DRD2	ADRA2B	5-HTTL-PR	MAO	TPH2	BDNF
Result	GG	AA	ID	SS	GG	GT	GG

The average person looks at this alphabet soup of letters, scrunches up their face, and says, "Huh?" However, a geneticist or functional genomics practitioner can look at these results and immediately understand how the results may impact your life.

When a practitioner does interpret your results, it's important to know that the insights they give you are associations, not diagnoses. Just because you are more or less inclined toward a predisposition does not mean that you *will* have that tendency. The same goes for the reverse. Diet, lifestyle, environment, family history, and your own personal past experiences all play a role in shaping your unique mood and behavioral profile as it is today.

Here are summaries of how my genome may impact various aspects of my life.

Work and Career

According to my genes, I am more likely to excel in reward-oriented careers such as sales, business development, and entrepreneurship. That's good because it's what I'm doing!

I have fairly "normal" proclivities in the following areas.

I am neither more nor less likely to be personally invested in or influenced by emotions in careers that involve high levels of trauma or stress or are tied to emotional situations. Examples of these positions include coroners, ER doctors, nurses, disaster crew members, first responders, paramedics, etc.

Likewise with investing; I can be an emotional investor or a logical, data-driven investor.

For example, in my business, I care deeply about the people we are helping to live better lives, but I need data to help me make decisions and chart a course for the future.

The same holds true for how I react to failure, disappointment, sorrow, and loss. My genes indicate I will neither overreact nor underreact. If a deal falls through, I'm not going to whimper and curl up in a ball under my desk, but if I close an important deal, I'm probably not going to do cartwheels around the office, either. Also, I'm not sure I can do a cartwheel.

I require, at the same rate as anyone else, novelty or constant challenges and changes in my work to prevent the risk of boredom in my work and career. For instance, I don't think I'd do well repeatedly doing the same task on an assembly line.

I'm likely to change positions or companies as much as the average person. Regardless of what their genes indicated, people used to spend their entire lives working for one or two companies. Those days are long gone, and I have proven that to be true in my own career.

I'll probably become distracted when completing a task—same as most people. So, if my son uses my favorite pen to pop a balloon next to my head while I'm trying to write this, I will likely jump in my seat, momentarily stop breathing, and stop writing.

If I am emotionally invested in and enjoying work, my performance is outstanding. That's understandable. I mean, who wants to take out the trash or mow the grass or do their taxes? I don't, and I'm not very good at doing any of those things. But if I'm selling something I believe in, I excel at it.

I'd prefer to work or complete tasks in "bursts" or "sprints" as opposed to working consistently over a specified period. Most people are like this, right? No one, not even a machine, can perform at 100 percent capacity 100 percent of the time and get good results. We too often treat ourselves this way. I know I did, and it nearly killed me.

Family and Relationships

I am more likely to have wider mood swings, become easily irritated, and make others conscious about their interactions—requiring what's sometimes described as "walking on eggshells"—around me. The fact that my genes indicate I'm likely to let my mood dictate my interactions in various relationships makes me wince. On the other hand, knowing this removes the character judgment I may place on this, and it gives me an opportunity to take steps to mitigate it in my life.

My genes indicate I will be influenced by and remember negative emotional events, such as arguments or fights, as much as the next person, but not more so, and not less. You may recognize this if you're arguing with someone, and they bring up something you said or did 20 years ago. Or if you ruminate on the time you were the only kid in your class not to get an invitation to a particular birthday party in fourth grade, your genetics say you're more likely to be influenced by these negative emotional events than the average person. According to my gene results, I'd probably be evenhanded should things like that happen to me, and I would likely forgive Anthony Goodrich, who was my dear friend at school and on our baseball team until he decided to swing his bat straight into my face.

My genetic capability to intuitively pick up on body language and facial cues is the same as the average individual. So, if a colleague at work grimaces and raises an eyebrow at one of my suggestions, I'm likely to notice it. The phrase "read the room" comes to mind here.

Finally, I have the same need to build strong emotional connections in relationships with friends and family as anyone else.

Diet and Nutrition

My genetic results suggest that I am more likely to use food as a coping mechanism for managing stress or negativity than the average person. Without knowledge of this predilection, I'd probably eat or drink something unhealthy—"comfort food"—to get through tough times. Given my genetic makeup, a better choice would be to meditate, listen to music, exercise, or do other healthy calming behaviors.

At the same time, when I do use food as a coping mechanism, I'm just as likely as anyone else to binge instead of grazing or snacking. This means that while I may want to eat macaroni and cheese if I'm crunching on a deadline and feeling stress, I'm neither more nor less inclined to want to eat an entire tub of it.

Sleep

Like many entrepreneurs, my genetic wiring makes sleep somewhat of a battlefield for me. This means I am more likely to stay up at night thinking about hypothetical situations such as an investor possibly dropping out, a product potentially being delayed, or any other of a million calamities. It goes with the territory, but I'm particularly inclined, from a genetic standpoint, to have difficulty with this.

In the same vein, I'm more likely to stay up at night thinking about conversations or interactions that happened throughout the day, as well as how the conversation could have gone either way.

Likewise, my genetic wiring suggests I am more likely to struggle to get rid of unhappy thoughts or unhappy memories when lying in bed than a person with "normal" genetic wiring.

The good news is, if I practice good sleep hygiene, I have the same ability as anyone else to achieve deep, rested sleep (even with seven to eight hours of sleep) and to fall back to sleep if I wake up during the night.

Pleasure

When Ovid, the ancient Roman poet, spoke about how anxiety is the flip side of pleasure, he could have added addiction, depression, stress, and burnout. I doubt people living in his time (43 B.C.–17 A.D.) had those words to describe the opposite of pleasure, but if anyone would have known them it would have been Ovid. Because while he was popular in his day writing about love, beauty, and seduction, Ovid was banished from Rome by Emperor Augustus to a remote province on the Black Sea at the age of 51, where he remained until his death. There, his writings turned to the topics of sadness, desolation, and despair over not being allowed to return.

Nineteen centuries later, when John Keats, the English poet, described pleasure, he said, "Give me books, fruit, French wine and fine weather and a little music out of doors, played by someone I do not know. I admire lolling on a lawn by a water-lilied pond to eat white currants and see goldfish: and go to the fair in the evening if I'm good."

Like Ovid and Keats, most people can describe what pleasure *feels* like, but they probably don't understand its biological basis. As in, scientifically, how does pleasure happen? Is there something going on in the brain? In your fingertips? On your tongue? Your nose? What about your eyes and ears? In the case of Keats, this is despite the fact that he was not only a poet but someone who studied science at King's College and trained to be a surgeon.

Reading this, you may recall Dr. Ruth Westheimer's catchphrase "If it feels good, do it," and wonder why you should care where pleasure comes from. You need to know because it has many implications for your health. In this section, we'll look at the flip side of pleasure—addiction, depression, stress, anxiety, and burnout.

First, let's state the obvious: pleasure is the response you feel when you do something enjoyable. Biologically, the pleasure response begins with a stimulus, such as a slice of your favorite cake, a sexual encounter, landing a business deal, or winning an award. And your biology determines how you respond to that stimulus.

Consider the following scenario.

Nicole and Anna are two sisters who go to an amusement park. When they arrive, they start talking about what to do first. Nicole only cares about getting on the roller coaster and doing the bungee jump. No other rides interest her. The faster and higher the roller coaster, the more fun she will have. She can't get enough of that feeling she gets in her stomach when the roller coaster drops. Anna hates roller coasters. She's convinced that the seatbelts on the roller coasters aren't properly installed and that she will fall out of the roller coaster.

The more they talk about the roller coaster, the more Anna starts to stress. She needs a distraction. Suddenly, Anna smells something delicious. The sweet, cinnamon smell of funnel cakes. Now, Nicole can't get Anna to do anything else. All this talk about roller coasters has stressed Anna out, and she needs something to make her happy. The only thing that will calm her down is funnel cake. So Nicole decides to go on a roller coaster ride while Anna eats her funnel cake.

There is no right or wrong in this scenario. There are two people, each with their own biology, responding to pleasurable stimuli in their own way.

In general, the pleasure response takes place in three phases.

Phase I is the anticipation phase. For example, think about your favorite food. Some people start salivating when they think about their favorite food, while others have no reaction until their favorite food is in front of them. The anticipation of doing or experiencing one of the above examples of stimuli causes your brain to release a chemical in your brain known as dopamine.

Phase II is the actual pleasure response itself, which only occurs after dopamine binds to receptors in a part of your brain known as the nucleus accumbens. This is when you are in the heat of the moment. It could be the minute you take your first bite of cheesecake or the moment your favorite team scores the winning goal. Until the dopamine binds to your receptors, you are in anticipation or Phase I mode.

Phase III is the aftermath of your pleasure response. This stage is characterized by how long or how quickly you return to a normal state of mind after experiencing pleasure. Some people live off their "high" for a long period of time, while others experience that feeling of pleasure as too fast for them to truly enjoy it, so they don't really feel any satisfaction.

The genes in your DNA play an important role in shaping your unique pleasure response. Specifically, genes in your DNA influence how long you stay in anticipation mode (Phase I), how intense your response is when you finally engage in the pleasurable activity (Phase II), and how long it takes for you to come back down from your pleasure "high" (Phase III). Naturally, these genes also influence feelings that are the opposite of pleasure, such as addiction, depression, stress, anxiety, and burnout. Considering the prevalence of these concerns in society today, let's take a closer look at them, using my own genome as an example.

Addiction

Addiction is a state in which a person chronically and compulsively pursues a reward or a practice that eventually becomes a habit. Addictive tendencies revolve around your relationship with pleasure. Meaning, a person can become addicted to almost anything because they feel pleasure while doing that act.

There are two types of addictive tendencies found in most people. These tendencies are influenced by the COMT and DRD2 genes.

The COMT gene controls how long you feel an emotion like pleasure. Are you more likely to think about something that makes you happy or is an emotion like pleasure just something you need to do and get out of the way?

The DRD2 gene controls how intense your pleasure response is. Are you more of a "go all in" kind of person or a "push yourself to the limit" kind of person?

Addiction Type 1: Reward-Based

These types of addictive tendencies are driven purely by a necessity to achieve pleasure.

Individuals in this category tend to display a behavior commonly described as "risk-reward" behavior. Because their anticipation and aftermath phases are shorter than normal, it takes a lot for them to get excited, and a lot for them to stay excited. They are generally described by their friends and family as thrill seekers and risk takers. For them, it is always about pushing the boundaries. They seem to crave higher and stronger pleasure responses because things that please others simply don't do it for them. These individuals, however, can also quickly turn toward harmful habits when they aren't challenged or driven by healthy opportunities. Addiction to pornography, alcohol, or illicit substances is often combined with feelings of depression, lack of purpose, and general lack of satisfaction unless they are involved in their activity of choice. These individuals often feel a need to frequently engage in their addictive behavior because they feel that they simply can't achieve pleasure without that experience.

Addiction Type 2: Bingeing

The second type of addiction focuses more on the intensity of the pleasure response.

Individuals with this type of addiction are blown away by the sheer joy they experience; they just cannot get enough of that feeling. They end up diving deep into that experience, often engaging in bingeing episodes. These people don't necessarily need pleasure every day, but they do occasionally go all out on their addictive behavior so they "get it out of their system."

The differences are subtle yet significant between the two types of addictions. The first type is driven by the desire to experience pleasure, while the second type is more about feeling the intensity of experiencing pleasure. A person with the first type of addictive tendencies may, for example, be addicted to drugs or alcohol in any form, while a person with the second type of addictive tendencies is only addicted to a specific type of drug or alcohol, say cocaine or whiskey. Recognizing the type of addiction an individual has can help personalize the recommendations they need since they will be different for each addiction type. Moreover, becoming aware of these tendencies and understanding the impact on their lives is always the breakthrough step toward any solution.

In my case, my genes indicate I am more likely to have the first, reward-based addiction.

This means my anticipation and aftermath phases are shorter than average, and it takes a lot more to get me excited and keep me excited. As a thrill seeker and risk taker, I may crave adrenaline-filled activities like skydiving, mountain climbing, roller-coaster riding, or even stock trading.

My test results indicate that I may also enjoy and engage in reward-based tasks or careers like entrepreneurship, sales, or business development. I may tend to jump from one activity to the next by becoming completely engrossed in new experiences while quickly becoming bored with the old ones. As a result, I am more likely to seek out that exciting feeling elsewhere, and that may include negative habits like drugs, alcohol, and gambling to get my "high," especially when I feel "unfulfilled" in my lifestyle or career.

Thankfully, while other family members of mine did succumb to destructive addiction, I channeled my genetic tendencies into less harmful and more productive activities.

If you take the stigma out of the word *addiction*, everyone has some form of addiction or behavior that isn't productive or helpful in their lives. An alcoholic may have a more severe form of addiction than someone who does something less destructive, but neither behavior is healthy. For instance, although I'm not an alcoholic, I've engaged in the more socially acceptable addiction of workaholism—and it has cost me.

Wherever you are on the scale of addiction, you should know that the highest highs don't have to be followed by the lowest lows. Instead, you can pursue pleasures that enhance your quality of life and have lasting, positive results.

When it comes to tackling unwanted habits, rather than just holding yourself to the "quit cold turkey" approach, you can create new habits, redesign your environment, and remove or reduce your dependency on pleasures that promote negative results.

Select those options that seem realistic in your life. And for addictive patterns that are harming you in substantial ways, please find a professional who specializes in that area.

Depression

Depression is a complex mental health disorder that often results from a combination of an individual's lifestyle, family history, environment, and genetics. Depression negatively affects how you feel, think, and act and can be described as prolonged feelings of sadness, loss, or anger. It can also be accompanied by physical symptoms such as fatigue, tiredness, and lack of energy. This section explores how genes can play an influential role in the development of some depressive tendencies in certain individuals.

In the section on addiction, I noted that consistently reaching a level of pleasure may not be easy depending on the versions of genes you carry.

Depressive symptoms typically described by some individuals include "a lack of purpose" or "a lack of a reason to get up in the morning." In other words, these individuals feel like they do not have anything that motivates them enough to get them going.

Individuals that fit into this category—like me—often do not achieve pleasure the way that other individuals do. They are often not satisfied with normalcy. They prefer to do things in extremes, pushing the bar or upping the ante in many aspects of their lives. Their idea of fun revolves around the concept of high risk, high reward.

People with these predispositions often thrive in high-pressure environments or careers, such as sales or entrepreneurship. When they are removed from the opportunity to engage in these environments, it is difficult for them to identify other avenues to achieve the same experience. As a result, they often experience feelings described as "something's missing." They are more likely to engage in addictive tendencies that offer them a false sense of achievement. These individuals tend to crave the pleasure response they experience when closing a sale, growing a business, or accomplishing a seemingly impossible task. As a result of the lack of a challenge or perceived pleasure, these individuals often display symptoms that are characteristic of depression.

I was one of them. And because I was sick and tired of being sick and tired, as in the case of addiction, I developed a list of things to do and not do. I didn't have to do all of them or even most of them. The idea was to start small, with achievable things, even if it was just one thing, and then build from there.

Taking small steps is important because depression can be debilitating. People in the grips of depression may not see a good path forward. They feel stuck—and unmotivated. However, there are simple and practical steps to help people with depression. These steps can start to alleviate the depressive moods and tendencies. A combination of daily physical activity, a diet of nutritious whole foods, and an optimized, regular sleep schedule can positively impact your overall level of depression. Along the way, you'll benefit from improved mood and biological processes like better skin, sleep, sexual health, and more.

There is no single solution for depression that works for everyone. You'll likely need to make a bundle of precise changes in your life. The challenge is to find which changes are best for you, which often involves a process of trying new habits without focusing on perfection. Instead, you are testing how changes work in your life.

And it all starts with understanding your DNA.

Stress

In 1936, Hans Selye, a Hungarian Canadian scientist at McGill University, became the first person to give a scientific explanation for biological stress. Until then, any understanding of stress was limited to the world of physics and the impact one object might have on another. Selye called his stress model general adaptation syndrome (GAS), a rather unfortunate acronym for such a solid bit of science. Based on physiology and psychobiology, GAS stated that an event that threatens an organism's well-being (a stressor) leads to a three-stage bodily response: alarm, resistance, and exhaustion.

Sounds harmful, doesn't it? It can be; if not understood it can cause a myriad of health problems. But as Selye also said, "Stress is the spice of life. It is not necessarily bad and depends on how you take it. The stress of exhilarating, creative and successful work is beneficial, while that of failure, humiliation or infection is detrimental."

Whether we avoid stress or court it for its positive properties, we are bound to encounter it every day of our lives. Consider the following scenario.

When they were young, it became clear to their parents that Anna and Nicole were different. One day, when their mother returned from a particularly rough day at work, having gotten into an argument with her supervisor, Anna and Nicole rushed to greet their mother and ask if they could eat the cookies she had baked the night before. Their mother, visibly still frustrated from her workday, brushed them off and asked them to clean their rooms first.

Anna, unaware of her mother's experience at work, immediately noted her mother's facial expressions and wondered if she hadn't greeted her mother in the way she liked. As their mother went to her room to unwind from the tough day, Anna and Nicole, being average eight-year-olds, simply went to the kitchen and started eating the cookies. When their mother came down, she lost her temper and shouted at both children, demanding that they go to their rooms for the rest of the night as punishment. Both girls went to their rooms, but one was clearly more affected than the other. Nicole quickly picked up that Mom was having a bad day and decided she would simply hang out in her room until Mom was feeling better. She knew her mother always came back and explained what was going on and that her mother loved her very much. On the other hand, Anna entered her room completely distraught. Negative thoughts flooded her mind, convincing her that her mother had finally grown tired of her and didn't love her anymore. Perhaps it was best that she simply run away.

When their mother eventually was able to relax, she entered each child's room and recognized the need to address what had happened in different ways for Nicole and Anna. For Nicole, it was simply a confirmation of what she thought. For Anna, it was important that her mother explain to her that it wasn't the child's fault, but rather the bad day that her mother had experienced before coming home.

All of us can relate to feeling stressed. It's a situation that triggers your body's natural response to physical, mental, or emotional pressure. As an entrepreneur, I feel stress every day, so I know it intimately.

Stress may also be our reaction to being put under pressure, making it difficult for us to cope with our demands. Each person responds differently to stress, but in general, the physical and mental symptoms of stress include raised blood pressure, increased heart rate, increased blood sugar, and acute feelings of frustration, sadness, anger, anxiety, and depression.

Stress isn't a bad thing all the time. The first day of a new job or the anticipation of a first date may be considered a good form of stress. However, stress should be temporary. Over time, chronic stress can be a significant contributing factor to many chronic diseases, including cardiovascular disease, obesity, hypertension, fatigue, anxiety, burnout, and depression. Your body's emotional response to stress plays a crucial role in your tolerance of external pressures. The interaction of specific genes influences your emotions and, as a result, can affect your stress tolerance.

Some stress is inevitable, and even helpful in the right time and place! But when stress is an ongoing, chronic condition of your life, take steps to address it to avoid the detrimental health effects associated with chronic stress. These steps will help make you more resilient to burnout by improving your physical, emotional, and mental capacity to meet the challenges in your life.

Let's look at some of the more harmful results of unmanaged stress.

Anxiety

The American Psychological Association defines anxiety as "an emotion characterized by feelings of tension, worried thoughts, and physical changes like increased blood pressure."

I can relate to this, because I have a moderate profile when it comes to my genetic predisposition toward feelings of anxiety. I'm close to the middle of the scale, leaning a little toward the problematic side.

We all get anxious from time to time. It's what rattles us before a big test and what makes our hearts beat a little faster before a presentation. But for people who live with anxiety, these feelings are much more than the everyday nervousness everyone feels. If you suffer from an anxiety disorder, these dreaded feelings continue to loom.

Anxiety sufferers typically report having recurring intrusive thoughts or concerns and experiencing physical changes like increased blood pressure. You may tend to avoid certain situations out of worry and may display physical symptoms such as sweating, trembling, dizziness, or a rapid heartbeat.

The COMT, DRD2, and ADRA2B genes influence your risk of developing anxiety symptoms. These genes layer upon and interact with one another to collectively trigger responses within your cells, influencing both the length and the intensity of your emotional response.

My genetic profile suggests I'm more likely to succumb to increased episodes and stronger feelings of anxiety. This means neurotransmitters like dopamine and noradrenaline tend to not linger long enough in my brain and create a heightened level of frustration in dealing with my emotional response. In addition, I may experience dysregulated serotonin reuptake, which is associated with wider mood swings and increased feelings of frustration.

This can often make it feel as if it is difficult to overcome the task, relationship, or obstacle in front of me, which can set off a chain reaction of negative feelings.

While it may seem logical to deal with anxiety in positive, constructive ways, it isn't always so. We think we're being weak if we even acknowledge our mood and behavior issues, so it's often difficult to actually work on them.

Anxiety is not only unpleasant, but it also may limit your ability to work, play, and connect fully with other people. In other words, anxiety can reduce the quality of your life and limit your potential. The good news is that you can manage anxiety better through changes in your habits and environment.

Burnout

Burnout is a chronic condition defined as "a state of physical, emotional, and mental exhaustion caused by excessive, prolonged, and repeated periods of stress." While anyone can experience burnout if they're subjected to enough stress, the capacity to manage and address causes of stress and reduce the risk of burnout varies among individuals. Your genes play an important role in defining this capacity.

Although I do not carry an increased likelihood for this health concern based on my genetic profile, I most definitely did become burned out. However, as I said earlier, just because I have a normal likelihood of burnout doesn't mean I won't become burned out if I make the wrong choices. I did, and I suffered the consequences.

An important gene in your DNA, the ADRA2B gene, controls your fight-or-flight response. That's the response that kicks in when your body is put into a stressful or negative situation. Examples of these situations might be an argument, road rage, a barking dog, a car crash, or an ugly breakup with a loved one. In each situation, noradrenaline binds to the noradrenaline receptor. The body activates a mode that causes physical and mental changes. Your muscles clench, your pupils dilate, your senses become more acute, and your brain processes information much faster.

The ON/OFF button of your noradrenaline receptor is controlled by the ADRA2B gene. When your body needs to enter a heightened emotional state as a response to an event, the receptor is turned ON by the gene and noradrenaline binds to the receptor to initiate the response.

Normally, the ADRA2B gene turns OFF the receptor, and the body quickly returns to a relaxed state once the negative moment has passed.

But for some people, like me, a deletion in their ADRA2B gene causes the receptor to stay ON for a longer time, resulting in the heightened emotional response staying activated for a longer time. This in turn results in prolonged hypersensitivity, particularly in response to negative situations. These individuals tend to hold on to negative events in their past and are easily reminded of those events if they are exposed to the right trigger. Over time, the continued existence in this state can significantly wear a person down, resulting in periods of burnout.

As I said earlier, before I got my DNA tested and began to understand why I was so sick, burnout was near the top of the list of things I experienced. When I asked how I could recover from burnout, my team gave me a series of recommendations. I didn't do them all, and I didn't do them all at once, but I have implemented many of them and they have helped me a great deal.

Calm and Chaos

The story of Dr. Deepak Chopra has always resonated with and inspired me. Early in his medical career, while practicing in India, he was focused on finding a biological basis for the influence of thoughts and emotions. After emigrating to the United States in 1970, he completed a residency in internal medicine, earned his medical license, opened a private practice specializing in endocrinology, and became chief of staff at New England Memorial Hospital.

In his 1991 book *Return of the Rishi: A Doctor's Story of Spiritual Transformation and Ayurvedic Healing,* Chopra wrote of his time as a hard-charging immigrant: "My days were blurring into nights. I was drinking black coffee by the hour and smoking at least a pack of cigarettes a day. I had acquired a taste for whiskey in the evening. My schedule kept my stomach upset all the time." He then recounts how, starting in 1981, he slowly became disenchanted with traditional Western medicine and began to incorporate more holistic methods of healing into his self-care, turning his life around. He was about 35 years old when he began his transformation, and since then he has become known the world over for his practices.

Aside from the cigarettes and whiskey, my immigrant family story is similar, albeit on a much smaller scale, including the tension between calm and chaos.

Let me try to explain the biological underpinnings of calm and chaos with the following scenario.

Jason and Michael are colleagues at the same financial technology start-up. Jason is a developer for the company's app, while Michael takes care of the company's marketing. They work together so that Michael's creative vision is appropriately presented in the company's app.

Jason often notes that while he's having a conversation with Michael, Michael frequently adjusts his own shirt, or fixes Jason's collar if it is off, or straightens a tilted portrait on the wall while they're speaking. He has also noticed that Michael becomes increasingly frustrated if Jason asks him to repeat his vision for the app they're developing a few times to make sure he understands correctly. For Michael, Jason feels it's all about doing things a certain way, and there's always resistance from Michael's end when it comes to trying out new things or ideas with the app. Michael has noticed that during meetings, Jason seems to be "not there" at times, as if he is thinking about other things. He believes that may be why Jason asks him to repeat things several times. He's also confused as to why Jason seems so relaxed about doing things on the go and not following the protocol of meeting > decision > action that they've developed in the company.

Michael's creative studio is best described as ordered chaos. He knows exactly where everything is, and he often gets upset when the cleaners come in the evenings and move things around while they are cleaning.

Jason often works remotely from his apartment. His workstation is empty except for his computer, and it faces a wall in the den of his apartment.

He prefers it that way, because the fewer distractions there are, the better. Jason has installed a focus app on his laptop, which only allows him a few minutes a day on Internet websites he enjoys, such as the news and gaming websites and social media. He also prefers to work during the evenings, as he can focus at night better than he can during the day.

The feeling of being calm or content may be hard to understand because most of the emotions we tend to feel either revolve around some degree of pleasure or its opposite, a lack of pleasure. In popular media, we are led to believe that being calm or content is synonymous with being happy. However, it is possible to exist in a state in which you feel neither happiness nor sadness. To be satisfied, in other words, doesn't necessarily mean to be happy. It simply means that you are not in a state of worry at the current time, but you are not necessarily in a state of happiness either.

Why are we going through the trouble of defining this feeling? It is important to understand that your ability to be in a state that is neither happiness nor sadness is critical in developing an ability to observe the world around you without bias.

A person who is constantly switching between happiness and sadness tends to look at the world through the lens of the feeling that they are currently experiencing. In both cases, there is a bias involved in how they view the world. It is also important to be able to evaluate what's going on around you and determine whether that thing is important to address, or whether it can be ignored or placed lower down on your list of priorities. Functional genes, particularly the genes that influence your relationship with the neurotransmitter serotonin, play a critical role in your ability to stay calm. Serotonin is often misunderstood as the "happy" neurotransmitter. While it certainly plays a role in achieving happiness, serotonin is more important for achieving an optimal balance between moods. Regulated serotonin binding helps reduce the risk of wide mood swings and maintain an overall calm state of being.

Let's examine a few health concerns that are influenced by your state of calm.

Empathy Versus Logic

When we look across the array of emotions and how people respond to situations, we observe a remarkable phenomenon. Some people seem to have a strong ability to show empathy and compassion, while others struggle to display socially acceptable empathy levels. Functional genomics offers a unique explanation for this phenomenon.

Deletions within the ADRA2B gene are related to our understanding of emotional sensitivity. They also play an essential role in your capacity for picking up emotional signals. In other words, a deletion in your ADRA2B gene can make it easier for you to pick up on facial, speech, and other social cues during an interaction.

You can also relate to another person's emotions because you have a strong connection with your own feelings.

This effect seems to be especially common in individuals with a slow COMT genotype, which breaks down the noradrenaline (a chemical messenger associated with fear, worry, and anxiety-based responses) that binds to the receptor (a docking station) to initiate the emotional response.

On the other hand, individuals with no deletion in their ADRA2B gene prefer to approach most situations with logic and rationality rather than emotion. What a person tells them is logically evaluated, analyzed, and then provided with a suitable response. This approach is often mistaken for being "cold," lacking sympathy, or simply not caring about one's feelings. However, the reality of the behavior is much more complicated. It is not that the individual is unable to have or show empathy; instead, it is how the person biologically processes emotional information and prepares a response. They may very well understand what someone is going through; they just don't display it as one might typically expect most people to respond.

Irritation and Frustration

While everyone gets irritated or frustrated, the tolerance that an individual possesses before they become irritated varies widely and depends on a combination of genetic and nongenetic factors. At the genetic level, individuals with a dysfunctional relationship with serotonin are more likely to have a lower tolerance toward irritation and frustration. In other words, things that would normally otherwise not bother the average person tend to annoy these individuals.

A variation in the 5-HTTLPR polymorphism located on your SLC6A1 gene, which controls serotonin transport, can cause serotonin reuptake to become dysregulated. Individuals that possess at least one S (or short) allele in this gene are more likely to have difficulty achieving a state of calm and are more likely to experience wider mood swings. They are more likely to struggle with prioritizing tasks based on their importance. They are also more likely to have a lower tolerance for irritation—in other words, they can become irritated far more quickly than the average person.

The TPH gene encodes the TPH2 enzyme, which is responsible for breaking down serotonin. Variations in this gene can influence the rate at which the enzyme breaks down serotonin. The faster the version of the enzyme (G/T and T/T genotypes), the less serotonin is available to bind to receptors and initiate its influence on your mood.

Let's run through two quick examples of genetic influences on irritation and frustration. Say you're explaining something to someone, and for some reason, they don't seem to understand you. The average person will likely attempt to explain it as many times as possible until the other person understands what they are saying. Those who have dysregulated serotonin, due to either a deletion in their 5-HTTLPR gene, a variation in their TPH2 gene, or both are more likely to become progressively visibly annoyed or frustrated the more they must repeat what they've said. Another example is when these individuals provide a specific instruction and that instruction is not carried out 100 percent as they have requested. These individuals are more likely to stress that the instruction must be 100 percent completed as they have requested rather than make concessions as long as the outcome is the same.

Irritation and frustration can cause anyone to become unhappy. These emotions, especially left unchecked, can also damage your personal relationships. What's less obvious is how irritation and frustration have a direct effect on your overall health and wellbeing. But the connection is there. These negative emotions can lead to reduced functioning of your immune system, cognitive processing, and more.

You can take action to change your habits and environment so you can benefit from better regulation of irritation and frustration. Even tiny steps can give big results.

Thinking Patterns and Neurotic Tendencies

The neurons in our brain are responsible for the transformation of information that forms the foundation of our mind. The way we think, come up with conclusions, are influenced by biases, and solve problems are all influenced by our neural connectivity. At the genetic level, a number of important factors that influence our thinking patterns are themselves influenced by variations within functional genes.

For instance, variations in your BDNF gene influence the levels of brain-derived neurotrophic factor (BDNF) produced by your body. BDNF is an important neurochemical found in your brain that influences the regions of your brain associated with eating, drinking, body weight, and mood balance. BDNF can influence your sleep cycles as well.

This factor is a crucial player in the "plasticity," or malleability, of your neurons. In other words, it influences how flexible your neurons are in forming new neuronal connections. This is important because individuals who have lower levels of BDNF tend to display similar or repetitive thinking patterns due to a more rigid neural connectivity. They often display a "hamster wheel" frame of mind, where they replay events or thoughts constantly, and they have difficulty seeing things in a different or novel light. This form of thinking can lead to the development of neurotic tendencies, where a person displays an irrational response to events that occur in their daily life. These tendencies can be further exaggerated if the person simultaneously has poor serotonin management, a heightened dopamine response, or hypersensitivity.

The A allele of the BDNF gene is associated with lower levels of BDNF and an increased likelihood of neurotic tendencies and repetitive thinking patterns.

People who have an increased genetic predisposition to specific thinking patterns and neurotic behavior should work toward supporting BDNF production to improve their quality of life. This has ramifications for your sleep and mental health.

In my case, my genes indicate I can display a mix of both empathy and logic, equal parts irritation and frustration, and "normal" thinking patterns and neurotic tendencies.

Of course, my optimal performance in this regard depends on the environmental, nutritional, and lifestyle loads I'm putting on those genes. Combine a negative circumstance in my life with not eating right, not getting enough sleep, and not exercising for a week and I can tell you with all certainty that I will be more chaos than calm, and I will not be at my best.

Focus

What I'm about to say is ironic and embarrassing, considering the topic of this section. As I was going through my notes to see what my research colleagues had written about the connection between our DNA and our ability to focus, I lost my focus. I wasn't mildly distracted—I was gone, at an I've-fallen-and-I-can't-get-up level of distraction.

Although I had blocked out the time to exclusively work on this book, before I realized what was happening, I was answering e-mails, taking phone calls, looking to see what the cause of some random noise was, checking social media, and going down a rabbit hole of statistics on the Web about how distracted we are and how much that distraction is costing us—financially, mentally, emotionally, and physically.

As a result, I was having an epic struggle with beginning this section. It's always hard to start something, but the more I distracted myself the harder it was to start. And the harder it was to start, the more I distracted myself!

I beat myself up for my shortcomings, telling myself I was weak and lazy and lacking discipline, which made it even harder. Although I am an avid reader of books and articles and research about self-improvement, focus, flow, mindfulness, and productivity, I began to question whether I had the credibility to say anything at all on this topic.

When I finally realized what was happening, I took a break from the computer. I put down my phone, exercised, took a hot shower, went outside, meditated, drank a healthy smoothie, and played on the floor with my son. In the process, I reset my system, regained my energy, and reclaimed my focus.

What do you imagine made me turn off the computer and get out of my self-destructive loop? I'll tell you—I reread the mood and behavior results from my genomic test.

As my results reminded me, based on my genetics, I am more likely than usual to lose focus when there is a distraction around me. Once I lose focus, it takes more time for me to get back to focusing on my task. Little things may annoy me a lot more than they annoy other people, such as a ticking clock, or someone who keeps interrupting me. When I add modern technology, my strong craving to satisfy my endlessly curious mind, and working from home into the mix, my distraction spreads like a wildfire.

I'm not alone. If you watch the film *The Social Dilemma*, in which Silicon Valley experts warn about the dangerous impacts of social networking, which Big Tech employs to manipulate and influence its users, you'll understand those companies are more than a little culpable for distracting us—it's part of their business model. Do the research yourself and you'll see, it's working.

According to a 2018 survey by Udemy, more than 70 percent of people say they are distracted at work. Attention spans are getting shorter and shorter. And, as I described with my own experience, it takes longer and longer to regain focus after you've lost it. In total, this lack of attention costs American businesses more than $650 billion per year. Moreover, it has a ripple effect on workers' lives. Thanks to being distracted, people are working longer hours to do the same work. With longer hours comes more stress. More stress brings more unhealthy habits. Unhealthy habits lead to poor performance, illness, and shorter life spans.

From a neuroscientific standpoint, when you're constantly losing focus you are weakening the physiological processes that ward off distraction. Conversely, the more you focus, the more your brain releases a chemical called noradrenaline, which aids in concentration.

So what do you do? There are plenty of suggestions available as to how you can fortify your ability to focus. For now, I'll point you to a book by Harvard-trained psychologist Daniel Goleman, *Focus: The Hidden Driver of Excellence*. In the book, Goleman explains that the prefrontal cortex of our brain, which controls executive functions such as concentrating, planning, and synthesizing, is in a continual battle with the more primitive part of the brain—sometimes referred to as the "lizard brain"—which controls our impulses.

I feel this battle whenever I sit in meditation. My prefrontal cortex sits quiet and undisturbed, while my lizard brain yells "squirrel" and takes off running like a hyperactive dog.

Once you understand that the job of your lizard brain is to make you jump at everything, you can tell it to quiet down. By working with your DNA, you can give yourself the best chance to make that happen.

The concept of focus is often used interchangeably with common terms and health outcomes such as ADHD, procrastination, distraction, and motivation, so let's look at it in those terms.

For this purpose, I will define *focus* as the ability to perform a specific task to its completion without conscious interference. In other words, how likely are you to complete the task at hand without being distracted, becoming bored by it, or resisting its undertaking or completion due to procrastination? I will also provide you with insight from a functional genomics lens, but it is important to remember that, like every other health outcome we evaluate, genetics is rarely the only cause or contributing factor.

ADHD

Attention deficit hyperactivity disorder is a medical condition generally characterized by difficulty in remaining still, impulsive behavior, a limited attention span, and a lack of attention to detail. Because of the wide variety of characteristics as well as the similarity of some of these characteristics to normal behavior, many children and adults are often misdiagnosed with ADHD. The clinicians who work with our researchers look at a patient's DNA test results and provide insights as to how functional genes play an important role in shaping the individual's focus and response, and ultimately how they potentially influence the person's ADHD-related tendencies.

A key aspect of understanding ADHD is understanding the influence of functional genes on the dopamine response. Specifically, how your COMT, MAO, and DRD2 genes influence the length and intensity of your dopamine response.

Let's walk through it together. Your COMT and MAO genes, as you read in an earlier section, influence how long dopamine stays available in your brain to bind to dopamine receptors.

Your DRD2 gene influences the density of your dopamine receptors. The lower the density of your receptors, the fewer receptors are available for binding and the less intense your dopamine response is. The faster your COMT and/or MAO enzyme, the less time there is for dopamine to bind to the receptor and initiate the response.

Individuals with this disposition are more likely to get easily interested in new things but will lose interest just as quickly once the novelty wears off or repetition sets in. Put simply, these individuals always need something new and exciting, something to change it up, to keep their attention and focus. When we look at a person with common ADHD symptoms, we can see how this starts to make sense. The lack of attention, of being "not there," or of trying to find something to physically do are all outcomes related to a need to experience the pleasure response that they are seeking.

As you know, ADHD can be disruptive to your home and work life. By increasing your ability to focus, you can set expectations and fulfill them more reliably. This not only will enhance your relationships at home and at work, but it also gives you greater confidence in your own capacity to set a goal and reach it efficiently.

There are many ways you can optimize your lifestyle to assist with improved focus and concentration. As the world gets more and more distracted by technology and on-demand sources of news, food, and digital media, it may feel like going against the current to create calm, focus, and moments for well-being.

Select a few one-time actions that can set you up for success, even when the pace of life feels fast and unfocused.

Procrastination

Procrastination can be generally defined as the act of delaying or postponing a task or series of tasks. There are many reasons why we procrastinate, and so trying to identify a singular cause or perhaps a singular set of functional genes that make you more likely to procrastinate is unlikely to yield accurate results. However, what functional genomics *can* offer is insight into the likelihood of contributing factors to procrastination as well as its auxiliaries: motivation and distraction.

Most people generally cite two reasons when it comes to procrastination. They either don't feel motivated enough to complete the task, or they experience anxiety at the thought of failing the task or facing the task itself. Both reasons can be, in part, explained by our genetics.

In general, individuals that show a greater likelihood of experiencing anxiety and hypersensitivity, most often associated with the *slow* version of their COMT gene and a deletion in their ADRA2B gene, are likely to exhibit procrastination due to a fear of failing at the task.

Individuals who display risk-and-reward patterns, generally classified by *fast* versions of their COMT and MAO genes, are likely to exhibit procrastination due to a lack of motivation or interest in completing the task. It simply does not excite them enough for them to want to engage and see the task through to completion. This includes me.

Distraction

In both cases of procrastination described in the previous section, your ability to respond appropriately to distractions can further influence your likelihood to procrastinate. Your brain's relationship with serotonin plays an important role in this phenomenon. Individuals who have a deletion in their 5-HTTLPR polymorphism tend to have dysregulated serotonin. This translates to an increased difficulty in classifying emotional stimuli based on their priority. Imagine that you are working on an important e-mail, and you notice the clock ticking. However, once you have noticed it, it becomes impossible to ignore unless you either move to a different room or take the clock dowh. Similarly, while having an important conversation with your partner, you may notice that the trash has not been taken out. Once you have noticed this, it becomes difficult for you to focus on the conversation because you want to make sure the trash gets taken out.

It's important to reduce procrastination in your life, because when you do, you will get more things done. But that's not all. You will have less guilt and shame about putting off tasks. Instead, you will complete tasks without a struggle, and you will feel good about your ability to get things done. This feeling will increase your confidence and abilities in other areas of your life.

As you can imagine, the number one piece of guidance could be "stop procrastinating." But we know that's not very helpful. Or realistic. Instead, at the end of this section, we've put together a short list of specific behaviors to stop.

Motivation

As I mentioned earlier, individuals with a *fast* version of their COMT and MAO genes and a *slow* version of their DRD2 gene often exhibit reward-seeking behavior. These individuals are motivated by the experience of pleasure they feel while completing a generally risky or challenging task. This may be identifying and investing in a high-risk stock before others, skydiving, or starting a successful business.

Believe it or not, fear is one of the most influential motivators most people possess. The fear of failure, fear of missing out, fear of what others will think, or fear of a decline in mental, physical, or material possessions are all common drivers of behavior. Individuals with a *slow* COMT, at least one D allele in their ADRA2B, and/or at least one A allele in their BDNF can all be significantly influenced by fear as a motivating factor for different behaviors.

The good news is that when you are realistic about how motivation functions in your life—and for human beings in general—you can be more compassionate with yourself and others. This helps you stop blaming yourself (and others) for lacking "willpower" or "discipline."

But that's not all. When you understand how motivation works, you can calibrate the difficulty of any task to match your current level of motivation. For example, if you're feeling super motivated one morning to tidy your house, then you can ride the motivation wave and tidy up a lot of things, maybe the entire house. In contrast, when your motivation sags the next day, perhaps you tidy up one thing and call it good enough.

In the next section, you'll find ways to understand motivation and apply those insights to optimize your life, as well as how you view the performance of yourself and others.

Mood and behavior form a critical part of our interactions with each other. Functional genomics provides insights into how these genes interact with each other as well as with our individual dietary, lifestyle, and environmental choices to ultimately shape our individual mood and behavioral profile. By understanding the influence of these genes, you should now have a much clearer and personalized route to achieving and maintaining an optimal profile. We strongly recommend that you discuss the tips, tricks, habits, and behaviors that we have recommended with your clinician or health care practitioner so you can build the personalized plan that works best for you.

STRESS

- Learn how to recognize physical signs of stress, like a sinking feeling, increasing blood pressure, hunching your shoulders, or a nervous tic.
- Reduce the people, activities, and contexts that cause you stress.
- Download an app that limits your use of social media.

- Make a list of things that cause you stress, both on a daily and a long-term basis. Get help with managing each of these stressors.

- Time management and organization are usual sources of stress. Use applications and take courses on how to effectively organize and manage your time.

- Put a pen and paper next to your bed and write down things that stress you at night. Promise yourself that you will review them in the morning.

- When you can't change your stressors, try changing the way you think about them.

- Increase your capacity to meet your stressors by focusing on your sleep, diet, and exercise.

- Talk to your boss about adjusting work demands to support your mental health. As a CEO, I don't have a boss, but I do have a board and advisors, and I talk to them regularly.

- Establish expectations for work and nonnegotiable time blocks in the evening.

- Visit a sauna a couple of times per week, especially if you have days that tend to be more stressful.

- When you come home from work, drink herbal tea like stinging nettle, chamomile, lemon balm, or lavender.

- Whenever you schedule a large project, block off a day or two after the final deadline to take a well-deserved break before you get pulled into the next project.

- Whenever you schedule a meeting, ask yourself if this could be a walking meeting where your colleagues join you outside, or you join by phone while you walk around your neighborhood or office building.

- Take supplements such as magnesium, vitamin B_{12}, ashwagandha, rhodiola rosea, and L-theanine.

ADDICTION

- Replace addictive junk food with nutritious snacks.
- Try monk fruit sweetener or stevia instead of sugar, which is highly addictive.
- Download an app that limits your use of social media.
- Block addictive websites on your browser.
- Replace pleasure with reward. Find something that gives you a sense of achievement.

Habits to Adopt

- Start your day like this: After your feet touch the floor in the morning, say, "It's going to be a great day."
- Buy nutrient-dense foods to feel full.
- Snack on dried fruit and nuts rather than candy.
- Always have a physical book or journal handy to read or write in.
- Open your watercolors, pick up your guitar, get out your chess set, or choose another hobby activity to participate in after dinner each night.
- Join a club or group that engages in a creative pursuit that you enjoy.

Behaviors to Avoid

There is no ideal way to stop all addictive behaviors. Each addictive pattern needs to be viewed on its own, in the context of the person doing the behavior. That said, here are some general behaviors I was advised to avoid:

- Purchasing unhealthy foods and drinks.
- Spending time with people who encourage unwanted behaviors.
- Having an alcoholic drink when you arrive home from work.
- Eating sweets immediately after you finish a meal. If you have to, set a timer and wait even 5 to 10 minutes.

DEPRESSION

- See a functional medicine doctor. There are answers other than pills.

- Take supplements: Studies have shown that some individuals experience improvement in depression symptoms after supplementing with vitamin D, high-dose omega-3, S-adenosyl-L-methionine (SAM-e), and magnesium.

- Start your day with time outdoors walking, jogging, breathing fresh air. Even sitting quietly in a nature spot can dramatically uplift your mood.

- Integrate physical activity into every day. Beyond fitness, think about adding movement throughout your routine to get more time outside and increase your baseline activity levels.

- Eat a diet rich in whole, unprocessed foods. Consider getting a meal-subscription plan that provides healthy, nutritious meals.

- Take a whole-foods cooking course to learn the basics of a nutritious diet. If you can't join a class, go to YouTube to watch videos on this topic.

- Make a list of nonwork activities you enjoyed in your past (such as painting or reading fiction). Bring them back into your life.

- Find a new challenge to channel your dopamine hit.

- Create a playlist of upbeat music that brings back the happiest times in your life.

- Make a list of the people that make you happy. Spend more time with them.

- Read daily from a print book that motivates you.

- Send a brief text message each day to someone who is positive and supportive in your life.

- Make "me" time a small but daily, nonnegotiable part of your life.

- Create a relaxing ritual each evening: Take a warm bath, relax in a sauna, do some gentle yoga, light a candle.

ANXIETY

- Avoid unnecessary situations and people who trigger your anxiety.
- Record instances where symptoms of anxiety occur and why you feel anxious about that situation.
- Realize that you are not alone: Many people struggle with anxiety issues. Find Facebook groups of people to support you.

Habits to Adopt

- When you notice anxiety in your body, set a five-minute timer and use that time to perform a breathing technique that addresses anxiety.
- Say a mantra when anxiety starts to build. For example, some people repeat this phrase attributed to Lady Julian of Norwich: "All shall be well, and all shall be well, and all manner of things shall be well."
- Attend a regular meditation class in person (or join one online).
- When you sense anxiety building, write down your concerns and worries. This type of journaling (sometimes called a "brain dump") is simple and effective for many people.
- Use anxiety-reducing techniques outlined by Dr. Ethan Kross in his book *Chatter*.
- Make herbal tea part of your daily life. Focus on lavender, chamomile, and lemon balm.

Behaviors to Avoid

- Drinking high-caffeine products.
- Relying on social media or the news to distract you.
- Maintaining relationships that are toxic for your mental health.

Supplements

- Deep Calm Optimizer
- L-theanine
- Ashwagandha
- Rhodiola
- Reishi mushroom extract

BURNOUT

- Talk to your boss about adjusting work demands to support your mental health.
- Use your genetic profile to understand how you think and what kind of work doesn't feel like work.
- Establish expectations for work and nonnegotiable time blocks in your evenings.
- Make a list of things that cause you stress, both on a daily and long-term basis. Think about how to get the outcome you need with a different process.
- Time management and organization are usual sources of stress. Take courses on how to organize and manage your time effectively.
- Put a pen and paper next to your bed and write down things that stress you at night. Promise yourself that you will review them in the morning.
- Identify toxic relationships and either address them or consciously choose to remove them from your life.

Habits to Adopt

- Learn how to recognize physical signs of stress, like a sinking feeling, increasing blood pressure, clenching your fists, or a nervous tic.
- Plan a visit to a sauna a couple of times per week, especially on days that tend to be more stressful.
- Brew herbal tea like stinging nettle, chamomile, lemon balm, or lavender when you come home from work.

- Whenever you schedule a large project on your calendar, block off a day or two after the final deadline to take a well-deserved break before you get pulled into the next project.

- Whenever you schedule a meeting, ask yourself if this could be a walking meeting where your colleagues join you outside, or you join by phone while you walk around your neighborhood or office building.

Behaviors to Avoid

- Buying junk food, which can reduce your ability to respond effectively to stress.

- Following multiple people on social media to get your news from and being overburdened with negativity—you don't need that stress.

- Always taking on tasks and requests and being unable to say NO—it takes practice to say NO more often, but it's a valuable tool to build!

Supplements

- Deep Calm Optimizer
- L-theanine
- Ashwagandha
- Rhodiola
- Magnesium bisglycinate
- Vitamin B_{12}

IRRITATION AND FRUSTRATION

Diet

- Increase your fiber intake by at least 20 grams a day with oats, flaxseed, beans, lentils, pineapple, plum, and cherry.

- Increase foods rich in chromium: broccoli, nuts, liver, plum, apple with the skin, beer yeast, whole grains, aged cheeses, mushrooms, spinach.

- Increase the consumption of foods that help promote serotonin: cocoa, banana, avocado, pumpkin seed, cherry, oats.

- Consume relaxing and calming teas: passion fruit tea, lavender tea, calendula tea.

Habits to Adopt

- Create a quiet workspace free of distractions. It may be helpful to turn your table to face the wall so you're not distracted by the outside world through your windows, but at least you still get some light into the workspace.

- Turn off (or minimize) notifications from your apps, your calendaring system, or your messaging platforms (such as Slack).

- Create a screensaver on your work computer that shows images of nature that help you feel calm (a tropical escape) or help you see the larger picture (a shot of the galaxy).

- Surround yourself at home and work with images that show people you love and scenes that help you feel calm and patient.

- Hire a meditation instructor to teach you loving-kindness meditation.

- Buy comfortable clothes and wear them when you work, especially on difficult projects (or with difficult people).

- Identify any tools in your life (from scissors to software) that cause you frustration. Then, purchase new tools that are easier to use.

- Meditate daily, especially the "loving-kindness" form of meditation.

- Whenever you are frustrated or irritated, say to yourself, "Everyone is doing the best they can. No one tries to screw up."

- Before entering a situation where you typically get frustrated (e.g., after you put on your seatbelt before your morning commute), set an intention to practice patience and kindness instead.

- At the moment you start to get annoyed, take three deep breaths to head off the escalation of that emotion.

- When someone begins to irritate you, try to take a comic perspective on the situation. Ask yourself, "What is funny about all this?" (There's almost always something.) Chuckle inside, if you can.

- When in periods of frustration and irritation (or immediately after), turn on a funny YouTube video or text an entertaining friend. Switch gears.

- Remind yourself that even though it makes sense in your head, what you say to others won't always click the first time they hear it. (A good way to practice may be to teach a child about something in the world, such as how clouds are formed, or how fish breathe underwater.) While it may feel frustrating at first, this practice will help you manage feelings better in the future.

- Learn how to temporarily step away from things that frustrate or irritate you. For example, if you're studying for an exam and you're struggling to understand concepts, step away for a little bit and drink a glass of water, stare outside, or go for a walk. Then come back fresh to tackle the task.

- When it comes to nutrition and emotions, focus your eating habits on fresh, nutrient-dense foods. Herbal teas are helpful as well, especially lavender, chamomile, and lemon balm.

Behaviors to Avoid

- Stop using social media during the workday. This includes YouTube. It's never "just five minutes."

- Stop making your phone easily accessible—put it in a different room or in a bag to reduce the urge to use it.

- Stop feeling guilty about getting distracted. It's only human. However, do take action to minimize distractions so you can stay focused.

- Stop scrolling on digital devices in the morning or evening. It can induce stress or distraction at the beginning and end of your day—both of which are the worst times for such things.

- Stop responding to e-mails in the middle of the night (distracting you from sleep and recovery). Instead, store your phone outside of the bedroom and set up an auto-reply after work hours.

Supplements

- Deep Calm Optimizer
- Magnesium bisglycinate
- 5-HTP (talk to your clinician before taking 5-HTP if you are on an antidepressant, particularly an SSRI)

PROCRASTINATION AND DISTRACTION

Habits to Adopt

- Redesign your physical environment to minimize distractions.

- Make it a habit to "just get started" on tasks you would rather avoid by scheduling them in your calendar.

- Learn to acknowledge when you are procrastinating and have a game plan to get you going on productive projects.

- Schedule pleasurable tasks around tasks you are most likely to avoid as a motivational tactic.

- Turn your phone on Do Not Disturb mode during eating, sleeping, and working times.

- Write down your top to-do list items after you sit down at your desk each day. Focus on the top three.

- Open any files/tabs for a work project that you're avoiding. Just write one line to make progress—even if that's all you do.

- Set timers for working on projects or tasks in chunks—15, 30, or 45 minutes at a time.

- If you really need a break, take it outside without any technology present.

- Do the easier parts of your tasks at the beginning of and after your breaks to help build momentum.

Behaviors to Avoid

- Using social media until the task at hand is done.

- Bringing your work into an ideation or personal space. Separate your "execution" space so you know it's time for work.

- Feeling guilty about getting distracted. It's only human. However, do take action to minimize distractions so you can stay focused.

- Scrolling on digital devices in the morning or evening. It can induce stress or distraction at the beginning and end of your days—both of which are the worst times for such things.

- Responding to e-mails in the middle of the night (distracting you from sleep and recovery). Instead, store your phone outside of the bedroom and set up an auto-reply after work hours.

Supplements

- Deep Calm Optimizer
- Acetyl-L-carnitine
- 5-HTP (talk to your clinician before taking 5-HTP if you are on an antidepressant, particularly an SSRI)

THINKING PATTERNS

Diet

- Increase the consumption of foods rich in DHA and ALA such as hemp seeds, nuts, flaxseeds, chia seeds, seaweed, and fish.

- Increase consumption of magnesium and B vitamins in foods such as lentils, peas, beans, oats, barley, avocados, bananas, salmon, and cashew nuts.

- Increase consumption of medicinal mushrooms such as reishi, lion's mane, and Cordyceps.

Habits to Adopt

- Follow a monitored exercise protocol—exercise boosts production of BDNF.

- Maintain a healthy, active lifestyle.

- Use a sauna often—sauna use boosts production of BDNF.

- Practice intermittent fasting.

- Set up a morning workout schedule—BDNF levels produced during the day help prepare the body for rest at night.

- Start you day with a hot shower—heat boosts production of BDNF.

- Turn your phone to Do Not Disturb mode after the workday is done.

Behaviors to Avoid

- Avoid the use of digital screens at night, which can disrupt your ability to fall asleep, particularly when the level of BDNF is already low.

- Avoid supplementation with pure S-adenosyl-L-methionine (SAM-e) to decrease the risks of neurotic behavior.

Supplements

- BDNF Optimizer

- Whole coffee fruit extract

- Magnesium L-threonate

A person's individual mood and behavioral profile is influenced by many factors, including diet, lifestyle, environment, family history, personal history, and genetics. At the biological level, our minds uniquely express emotions, memories, thoughts, and feelings depending on the important relationship between the neurochemicals our bodies produce, such as dopamine, serotonin, and BDNF, and the cells in our brain, known as neurons.

The genes in your DNA play an influential role in how these neurochemicals interact with your brain and ultimately influence your overall mood and behavioral profile. It is important to note, however, that the influence in the genes discussed here is not diagnostic but associative. In other words, while these genes may indicate a predisposition toward certain behaviors, the reality is that factors like diet, lifestyle, family history, personal history, and the environment can and will interact to dampen or augment the influence of these genes on your overall mood and behavior.

With that in mind, the suggestions I've shared with you can offer some notable insights as to how I am supporting my genes so I can have positive mood and behavioral outcomes. These insights are the result of prior published research as well as our own proprietary data analysis of over 7,000 genomic profiles from around the world. Keep in mind that I didn't share suggestions for some things, like ADHD and empathy versus logical thinking, because my results are optimal in this regard.

When you get tested and get your own suggestions, they will look something like what I've shared—but they will be personalized for *you*.

Chapter 5

DNA, DIET, AND NUTRITION

Ninety percent of the diseases known to man are caused by cheap foodstuffs.

— Victor Lindlahr, nutritionist and author of *You Are What You Eat: How to Win and Keep Health with Diet*

You know the saying "You are what you eat"? It's true in the sense that the structure, function, and health of every cell in your body operates on a foundation of the foods we eat.

Unfortunately, much of what we currently eat consists of food-like substances that are engineered by corporations, that are filled with ingredients we've never heard of and can't pronounce, and that prioritize profits over people and the planet. While our food should be dense with nourishing nutrients that help us prevent disease, lengthen our lives, and perform at our best, they are largely devoid of anything that even vaguely resembles the whole foods we should be eating. As a result, the foodlike substances we ingest are making us sick, unnecessarily shortening our lives, and causing us to underperform—that is, except for the food conglomerates who happily rake in billions of dollars for their efforts.

Although what I've described is dire, the good news is we know how to change it. The answer is in the recipe our DNA has laid out for us. I'm not talking about the DNA we've inherited from our parents, grandparents, or great-grandparents. I'm talking about our ancestral DNA from 250,000 years ago.

Before people learned how to farm around 10,000 years ago, humans got their food by hunting, gathering fruits and nuts and vegetables, and fishing. They ate what was available, season by season, getting enough nutrients to sustain themselves and thrive. The origin of their food sources was natural. For instance, if they had chickens, the birds generally weren't for eating; they were for laying eggs. But when the chickens were going to be eaten, they ranged free and feed on grass, like they were meant to. This meant they were healthy and produced healthy eggs. Today, because chickens are crammed into cages and stuffed with who knows what, they are now under great stress, their hormones are out of whack, and they are about four times the size they used to be. The eggs they produce look and taste artificial, and although the chicken is larger, it does not have the same quality or density of nutrients that ancient chickens did.

Bread is another example. Our ancestors relied on only a few grains, and when those grains were used to make bread, what resulted was a hard brick, again, dense with nutrients. As Andrew Weil has said of the era's bread, "If you could squeeze it, something was wrong." As the world's population grew, so did our need to feed all of those people. A few ancient grains became 10,000 soft, glutenous grains that had preservatives, that could resist pesticides and be stored for longer periods of time, and that even rats didn't eat.

I could repeat this scenario of short-term expedience for long-term loss for almost any food source—the humble potato used to be the size of a golf ball, for instance, and it had enough nutrients to be a meal all by itself—but you get the idea. I encourage you to read about the history of diet and nutrition as I have, and to watch the documentary *The History of Food*; it's fascinating and eye-opening.

For now, I'll say that we need to eat in a way that is more in line with how our ancient ancestors used to eat. That doesn't mean we have to run around with loincloths and spears to eat right, but our ancestors can teach us a lesson. Because of their nomadic, foraging lifestyle and ancient diet, they didn't develop high blood pressure, diabetes, cardiovascular disease, cancer, or most of the other ills that plague us today.

The truth is, our genes still haven't had enough time to adapt to farmed foods, and until they do, we can follow the recipe our DNA wrote for us.

Diet and nutrition form a complex, multifactorial system that is significantly influenced by the genes you carry in your DNA. By understanding the roles that the genes in your DNA play, as well as how variations in these genes can influence dietary outcomes, you can get sound, scientifically supported recommendations based on our current understanding of your genes and the nongenetic factors in your life—including the foods you choose to (and not to) eat, the lifestyle you live, and the environment in which you live.

Also, please remember, you should always discuss your dietary goals with a health care practitioner before embarking on any dietary or nutrition protocol.

By testing and evaluating variants within the COMT, DRD2, ADRA2B, 5-HTTLPR, MAO, FTO, and MC4R genes we can see what, when, and how different individuals should be eating. We can throw out all the fad diets and food myths and rely on hard science. No one-style-fits-all approaches. Instead, it's *your* style for *you*.

When I got my own DNA results, I had to make some changes. I can't tell you what you'll have to do because I don't know your DNA and the food choices you make. But I can share my own results and what they mean to me.

I learned, among other things, that an optimal diet and nutrition profile goes beyond simply *what* I eat. In fact, it has a lot to do with *how* I eat, *when* I eat, and *why* I eat. My mood, behavior, and personality all play important roles in my diet and nutrition choices. They do in yours as well.

Here's an overview of my genomic tests for diet and nutrition:

Gene Tested	COMT	DRD2	ADRA2B	5-HTTL-PR	MAO	FTO	MC4R
Result	GG	AA	ID	SS	GG	TT	CT

COMT, DRD2, and MAO

Your COMT, DRD2, and MAO genes all play a role in your overall pleasure profile. Pleasure is strongly linked with diet and nutrition because it can influence inhibition, control, diligence, and reward-seeking behaviors.

ADRA2B

Together with the COMT gene, your ADRA2B gene influences your emotional state, which can play an important role when it comes to diet and nutrition. Your emotional state can influence the dietary and lifestyle choices you make during periods of emotional duress, calm, stress, anxiety, or anger.

5-HTTLPR

Your 5-HTTLPR gene influences your serotonin transport and reuptake. Serotonin plays an important role in mood balance as well as eating and drinking behaviors. Individuals with certain variations in this gene are more likely to use food as a coping mechanism for the stress in their lives, which can impact their dietary choices during stressful periods.

FTO

Your FTO gene influences how efficiently your body communicates with your mind that you have achieved satiety.

It is important to understand the difference between satiety and satisfaction. Satiety is the state of fulfillment—your stomach communicates with your mind that you have reached capacity and don't need to eat anymore.

Satisfaction is the state of feeling you experience when you are satisfied. Instead of a physical change like in satiety, satisfaction occurs directly in the mind and does not always correlate with satiety.

MC4R

Your MC4R gene plays an important role in managing your hunger cues. It has a central role in energy homeostasis and somatic growth and is one of the most studied genes in relation to weight gain, particularly early-childhood weight gain. MC4R is primarily expressed in the hypothalamus region of the brain, the region of the brain that controls hunger and appetite. Genomic variations in the MC4R gene have been shown to play an important role in appetite regulation and hunger cues.

My Genetic Results and Behaviors

Like the average person, knowing that I'll eat my favorite meal later is enough to lift my spirits. Do I love my Thai food? Yes, and I look forward to eating it. But I have to be careful because my genes indicate I will go to great lengths to satisfy my food cravings.

My genetics say I'm not likely to overindulge at buffets or when eating that Thai meal. However, I am more likely to overeat after breaking a fast. Although I will generally be able to acknowledge when I've reached satiety (feeling full), like most people, I can have bingeing episodes from time to time with my favorite types of food.

I am not a particularly emotional eater. Some people turn to sweet, salty, or fatty food if they're feeling down. That's usually not the case with me. On the other hand, I am more likely to rely on food as a coping mechanism when I'm experiencing stress or anxiety. I'm also more likely to snack or graze throughout the day.

Based on my genetics, I have a tough time sticking to certain diets. It's not as much of a problem now, because I understand what my DNA is telling me and take corrective actions.

Food Sensitivities

Insulin

I am more likely to be resistant to insulin, which can contribute to an increased risk of type 2 diabetes. Insulin is the hormone that is released by the body in response to sugars in your bloodstream. Sugars can come from the breakdown of either fats or sugars. When you have an elevation in your blood sugar following a meal, insulin acts as a signal to your body to store any excess glucose in the liver until the sugar level comes down.

The efficiency with which your body responds to the signals of insulin is influenced by your TCF7L2 gene. Variations in this gene can determine how well your body responds to the presence of insulin and as a result, how well your blood sugar level is addressed. Genetic variations in TCF7L2 are associated with increased risk of insulin resistance and type 2 diabetes.

The G/G genotype is associated with normal insulin function and a reduced risk of type 2 diabetes. Individuals with this genotype will respond better to dietary interventions and restrictions (diets).

The G/T genotype is associated with dysregulated insulin function as well as an increased risk of insulin resistance and type 2 diabetes. Individuals with this genotype generally will have a poor response to dietary interventions and restrictions.

The T/T genotype—which I have—is associated with dysregulated insulin function as well as an increased risk of insulin resistance and type 2 diabetes. Individuals with this genotype generally will have a poor response to dietary interventions and restrictions. For me, this means I should limit sugar consumption (as well as fat consumption if you have an A/G or A/A version of the APOA2 gene) to reduce my risk of insulin resistance as well as of type 2 diabetes. However, any diet that is developed for individuals like me should acknowledge that too many restrictions will reduce compliance and likely increase the risk of bingeing or excessive cheat days.

In addition, individuals with the T allele will have a greater risk of cardiovascular disease due to the potential of elevated blood sugar levels as a result of insulin resistance. Sugars are inflammatory agents.

Gluten

I am more likely to have a normal response to gluten in my diet, with a moderate risk of gluten sensitivity. My risk is not necessarily due to the gluten itself but more to do with what is found on the gluten molecules, such as pesticides and herbicides.

Gluten is a structural protein complex contained in wheat and other cereals. Gluten is composed of two components: gliadin (a water-soluble component) and glutenin (a water-insoluble component). This bimorphic feature is what allows gluten to take on its sticky and chewy characteristic when mixed with water. The gliadin component of gluten elicits the strongest autoimmune response.

Gluten-related disorders include three distinct subgroups.

Celiac disease, which is when a genetic predisposition triggers an autoimmune reaction to the metabolite of gliadin whenever gluten is introduced into your body. This is a clear and identifiable response.

Non-celiac gluten and wheat sensitivity, which is when an innate immune response to a yet-to-be-identified antigen (in other words, not the metabolite of gliadin as in celiac disease) combined with the response from your gut microbiome causes symptoms similar to those in celiac disease, but not always as severe.

Wheat-associated allergy, which is when a wheat allergy is a bona fide immunoglobulin response to wheat and is not the same thing as celiac disease or non-celiac gluten sensitivity.

One interesting question we've found is why do so many individuals suffer from non-celiac gluten intolerance when consuming U.S. or Canadian wheat, but not when consuming EU or UK wheat?

The answer likely lies at the intersection of the quality of wheat and your genetics beyond the typical HLA genes that we look at when trying to diagnose celiac disease. When compared to US/Canadian bread for example, EU/UK bread products are often lower in gliadin and are significantly less exposed to various glyphosates and other herbicides and pesticides.

In addition, your anti-inflammatory capacity influences your risk of gluten sensitivity. Genes like the GST family of genes, your FUT2 gene, and your vitamin D family of genes all play a role in your response to the chemicals and preservatives found in gluten-based products, particularly in North America. Many cultures around the world produce bread and other wheat products without preservatives that are meant for consumption on the same day. Therefore, eating bread loaded with preservatives can cause a reaction that many may confuse with gluten sensitivity.

Lactose

I am more likely to be lactose intolerant and will respond poorly to lactose in my diet.

Lactose is the major sugar found in cow's milk, but—depending on your genetics—you may not be able to digest it. It is formed through the bond of a glucose and galactose molecule. The body uses an enzyme called lactase to break down lactose into the two useable sugars. Historically, and relatively speaking, humans did not drink cow's milk until fairly recently. As a result, most humans are naturally lactose intolerant. However, in some areas of the world, humans have evolved at the genetic level to become more lactose tolerant.

Microbiome

I am more likely to have a weakened and susceptible microbiome profile.

An optimal gut microbiome is an important part of a good diet and nutrition protocol. There are several gene pathways that influence the strength, stability, and diversity of your gut microbiome. A rich and diverse gut microbiome promotes health and prevents chronic diseases. In contrast, poor diversity of the gut ecosystem is a characteristic feature of chronic diseases, including obesity, diabetes, asthma, and gut inflammatory disorders.

My FUT2 gene function performs very well as it relates to its impact on gut bacteria diversity and behaviors. On the flip side, having this profile makes me a poor absorber of vitamin B_{12} through my gut. To counteract my low vitamin B_{12} levels (because it's not being properly absorbed), I take vitamin B_{12} sublingually (dissolved under my tongue). The sublingual route bypasses the first-pass metabolism and facilitates more rapid absorption of the B_{12} into the systemic circulation through the blood vessels.

Unfortunately, I carry a suboptimal profile when it comes to the other genes that influence my microbiome. This means I am more likely to have a weakened and susceptible microbiome. For instance, via the glutathionization pathway, my GSTT1, GSTM1, and GSTP1 genes do not do a good job of influencing my body's ability to metabolize toxins that can harm my microbiome. In addition, via the vitamin D pathway, my CRP2R1, GC, and VDR genes are suboptimal in the way they influence the upregulation of protective mechanisms that guard the gut microbiome.

I guarantee I would never have known about my food sensitivities or the condition of my microbiome—or even that such things exist—without getting my genome tested. Unless you're a clinician or scientist you wouldn't be expected to know. However, like me, you are someone who can become an active participant in your own health and protect your microbiome through proper dietary, lifestyle, and environmental interventions.

Macronutrients

Try to watch television or look at your cell phone without seeing an advertisement that promises if you buy their product, you'll lose fat, gain muscle, have more energy, and more. There is a consistent barrage of sales pitches for powders, pills, drinks, dissolving tablets, and meal plans for keto, low fat, low carb, vegetarian, vegan—virtually every style of eating imaginable. Most of them focus on your appearance and say nothing about the bodily systems and genetics, not to mention your environmental, diet, and lifestyle loads that are underpinning it all. When the only effort most of them require is you reaching for your credit card, you know there's a problem.

What if, instead of living to fit into our *jeans*, we lived in a way that fit with our *genes*?

We can do that by getting our DNA tested.

Here's an overview of how my genetics relate to different types of diets that are being pushed today:

Gene Tested	HLA rs2187668	HLA rs7454108	HLA rs2395182	HLA rs7775228	HLA rs4713586	HLA rs4639334
Result	AC	AA	CC	GG	CT	TT

Low-Carbohydrate Diets—Like Keto

Carbohydrates are a major source of energy for humans. The major building blocks of all carbohydrates are known as monosaccharides. Monosaccharides are commonly referred to as simple sugars. Examples of monosaccharides include glucose and fructose. Two monosaccharides combine to create a disaccharide such as sucrose (or table sugar).

Multiple monosaccharides can form what is known as a polysaccharide. One of the most abundant forms of polysaccharides are starches, which are found in vegetables, including potatoes and rice.

Functional genes can influence your ability to break down various types of carbohydrates, including starches, sugars, and fibers. My DNA tests evaluated these genes' influence on my overall diet, nutrition, health, and wellness.

Here's what I discovered:

Based on my genetics, I would benefit from having a low-carbohydrate diet that integrates low levels of starchy carbohydrates.

Because I have an increased likelihood of gaining weight if I eat foods like rice, pasta, and breads, I should avoid them. No more than 15 percent of my carb intake should be from starchy sources, and *at least* 85 percent of my carb intake should be from vegetables and other fiber sources.

I carry a suboptimal insulin-sensitivity profile and have an increased likelihood of developing hyperglycemia (elevated blood sugar) particularly on a diet high in starches. This means I should avoid processed or added sugars in general and moderate my fruit consumption. Specifically, I should eat fruit in moderation, and be careful of overconsuming it, particularly at night, as the high sugars in many fruits can further disrupt my insulin-resistance profile.

My genes indicate that I am lactose intolerant. As a result, I should consider nondairy or lactose-free alternatives for milk, cheese, yogurt, and other dairy products I enjoy.

In terms of celiac or non-celiac gluten sensitivity, I am normal. This means I am more likely to have an average response to gluten in my diet, with a normal risk of gluten sensitivity. The risk I have is not necessarily due to the gluten itself but has more to do with what is found on the gluten molecules, such as pesticides and herbicides.

Low-Fat Diets—Like Vegetarian or Vegan

Fat is an indispensable building material for every single cell. It serves as the primary energy reserve in humans and animals. There are two major types of fats: unsaturated and saturated fats. The difference between them has to do with chemistry, but the outcomes are what is important. The third type of fat, which is not commonly found in nature but is highly prevalent in processed foods such as margarine, is called trans fat. There is unanimous support that trans fats are the most detrimental type of fat for the human diet. As a result, they should be avoided whenever possible. The type, amount, and version of fats best for your diet depends on several factors, including your unique genomic profile.

Here's what my genetic tests revealed regarding fats:

With suboptimal results in this area, it would be best if I have a diet that integrates low levels—no more than 10 percent of my daily intake—of dietary fats.

Because my genetics indicate I have an increased probability of developing hyperglycemia (elevated blood sugar) and gaining weight if I eat saturated fats such as butter, ghee, and cheese, I should keep them to a minimum under the watchful eye of a trained health care provider.

Since I do need some fat consumption as part of my diet, I should incorporate the following optimal fat sources: olive oil, avocados, nuts, and seeds.

The good news is, with a normal genetic ability to feel full and not overeat during my meals, I have a reduced risk of developing obesity.

High-Protein Diets

Unlike dietary fats and carbohydrates, there aren't variations in genes that influence protein metabolism. But we can evaluate how you respond to toxins found during the production and preparation of proteins, as well as the source of that protein. In this regard, I am highly sensitive to toxins. With that in mind, I have to avoid charred, burned, and smoked meats; eat up to one serving of grass-fed red meat per week; ensure I get one or two servings of fatty fish a week, choosing smaller fish like sardines, anchovies, or mackerel over larger fish like salmon or tuna; and do my best to avoid precooked or left-over meat, as the histamine content increases once a meat has been cooked—this is especially important for those with allergies.

Micronutrients

Can something that sounds so small have a big impact on our lives? Yes, far more than you may realize.

Large amounts of macronutrients, such as fats, carbohydrates, and proteins, when combined with small amounts of micronutrients, such as vitamins and minerals, keep every cell and system in your body working properly, including your immune system.

Much has been written about what micronutrients are and how you can get them through diet and supplements, including by Dr. Joel Fuhrman. I encourage you to do your research. Dive in, as I did, and read everything.

What I'm going to do is briefly talk about how your body may or may not be genetically equipped to handle micronutrients, as I did with macronutrients, again using my own results as an example.

Specifically, we will look at how my genes influence my ability to efficiently utilize vitamin A, vitamin C, zinc, and vitamin D.

Here are my results:

Micronutrient	Vitamin A BCMO1	Vitamin C SLC23A1	Vitamin D CYP2R1	Vitamin D VDP/GC	Vitamin D VDR	Zinc SLC30A8
Result	AG	GG	AG	CC	CT	AA

Vitamin A

My vitamin A results are normal.

Vitamin A is a fat-soluble vitamin that is found in many plant- and animal-based foods. The plant version is known as beta-carotene, while the animal version is known as retinol or retinyl palmitate. Vitamin A plays an important role in the health of your vision, immune system, and reproduction. Low levels of vitamin A can thus be a significant risk factor in many health concerns.

Beta-carotene must be converted into retinol before the body can use it. An important gene in your DNA known as BCMO1 produces the enzyme that facilitates this reaction. Beta-carotene oxygenase 1 (BCMO1) is an enzyme that plays a key role in the conversion of vegetable-derived beta-carotene (the inactive version of vitamin A) into retinol, the active form of vitamin A (usually derived from animal sources). Variations in the BCMO1 gene influence your body's ability to convert beta-carotene into retinol.

Vitamin C

My vitamin C results are normal.

Vitamin C is a potent antioxidant that acts as a scavenger in your body and hunts down oxidants (also known as free radicals). Humans do not naturally produce vitamin C, so they rely solely on dietary or supplementary sources for their daily intake. However, a specific family of proteins directs the absorption and distribution of vitamin C throughout your body.

A gene known as SLC23A1 determines the efficiency with which the proteins carry out this operation. As a result, variations in the SLC23A1 gene influence your ability to transport vitamin C effectively throughout your body.

Vitamin D

My vitamin D results are suboptimal.

The CYP2R1 gene encodes the enzyme responsible for converting vitamin D_2 into activated vitamin D_3. Variations in the CYP2R1 gene influence your body's ability to convert vitamin D_2 (absorbed from sun and diet) into vitamin D_3 (the active form).

The VDBP/GC gene encodes the vitamin D binding protein (VDBP), which is responsible for the binding, solubilization, bioavailability, and transport of vitamin D. It is the major vitamin D transport protein in the blood. Therefore, variations in GC influence the levels of vitamin D in blood plasma.

The VDR gene encodes the vitamin D receptor, which is responsible for binding with vitamin D and initiating the associated functions of vitamin D. It plays an important role in the VDR transcriptome, which influences the efficiency of the body's overall immune system. Variations in the VDR gene influence the efficiency with which vitamin D binds to the receptor and exerts its intended influence.

Because my body does not efficiently activate, transport, and/or bind vitamin D to its receptor, I take an increased-dosage vitamin D protocol and split my dose into a morning and afternoon serving so my levels are more consistent throughout the day.

Zinc

My zinc results are suboptimal.

This means I am more likely to have higher fasting and post-prandial (in the period up to four hours after eating a meal) glucose levels. Since I do not efficiently bind and transport zinc in the beta cells of my pancreas, which may result in reduced insulin crystallization and activation, I take a daily zinc dose of 14 mg.

Zinc is an essential trace mineral necessary for the human body in small amounts and it cannot be naturally produced by the human body. As a result, humans rely directly on dietary and supplementary sources of zinc for their daily intake.

Zinc is required to complete several important processes in your body, including gene expression, DNA synthesis, optimal immune function, sugar management, healing of wounds, and your body's overall growth and development.

When it comes to the way your body deals with sugars, zinc plays an important role in activating insulin. In order to activate insulin, which is released from the pancreas in the presence of sugars in your bloodstream, zinc must be transported through your cells to begin the activation process.

An important gene known as SLC30A8 encodes the protein that transports zinc to the appropriate site of action in your cells in order to activate insulin. Variations in this gene can influence the efficiency with which zinc is transported, which can impact how quickly insulin is produced in response to an increased level of blood sugar. As a result, zinc levels play an important role in managing your risk for type 2 diabetes.

When I first looked at the report my colleagues gave me about how my genetics influence my diet and nutrition, I was enthusiastic. I finally had some insight into why I was feeling and behaving the way I was.

Then I got to the part about changes I'd have to make if I wanted to heal myself and live longer with more vitality. That's where the hard part comes in. Because although we *intend* to make healthy choices, we all know what that road is paved with and where it's headed. Actually making healthy choices is hard, particularly when unhealthy choices always seem to be within arm's reach.

If I knew anything, it was that a positive attitude helps everything. What I didn't know was that my belief was supported by a recent study published by the journal *Appetite*, which found that a positive attitude helps in eating healthy.

The study looked at what motivates people to learn about nutrition and incorporate healthy food into their lives. Taiwan, where the study was conducted, used to be a healthier country, but it has seen steadily increasing rates of obesity, high blood pressure, and diabetes due to poor dietary habits. Researchers in the study asked participants about their approach to learning about nutrition and making changes.

The findings suggest that when it comes to influencing behavior, there is a wide gap in effectiveness between people who pursue health versus those who want to prevent illness. In practical terms, that's the difference between someone who wants to live a long, healthy, and vibrant life, and someone who's afraid of dying young due to some disease.

While the second mildly concerns me, I am without a doubt in the first camp. That's why I have incorporated most of the recommendations that were made for me and that I'm about to share with you.

Please understand, these are the recommendations that were made for *me* when I began *my* journey, and they're based on *my* unique genetics. Once your genome is tested and analyzed, then you can decide whether or not you'll act on the recommendations you'll receive. And, as always, you'll need to make those decisions in coordination with your doctors.

I share these recommendations with you to show what I did, and continue to do, based on the results of my genetic tests in several areas.

Overeating

- Avoid buffets and all-you-can-eat restaurants.
- Drink a glass of water mixed with a little apple cider vinegar to help curb your hunger and induce satiety.

- Eat something small before going to social events with food.
- Create variety for your palette to increase satisfaction.

Emotional Eating

- When you are upset, you will look for something to cheer you up. This is true for anyone with the L/S or S/S 5-HTTLPR gene. Try something other than food, such as traveling, going for a walk or a drive, working out, meditating, or reconnecting with an old friend to help you get out of your emotional state.
- Set up your favorite meals as rewards on specific days when you have a number of tasks or chores to complete to turn it into a rewarding experience.

Snacking and Grazing

- Eat nutritionally dense meals—by eating the rainbow as well as a combination of different flavors, textures, and sensations, you are less likely to want to satisfy other cravings throughout the day.
- Avoid keeping junk food in the house and replace it with healthy alternatives, such as carrots instead of potato chips, hummus instead of fatty or creamy dips, and more than 70 percent dark chocolate instead of store-bought sweets.

Bingeing

- Bingeing can be therapeutic if done right.
- Buy the most expensive and smallest version of your favorite ice cream or binge food.
- Allow yourself to binge once a month after you accomplish difficult or boring tasks.

Sticking to Diets

- Change the way you look at the diet—it's not just temporary, it's permanent! Plus, you're not only losing pounds, you're gaining health!
- Don't put too many restrictions on food right from the start—grow yourself into the diet.
- Start with trying the diet out a few times a month, then once a week, then every other day.
- Slowly take out things from your diet one at a time.
- Watch videos on how to cook healthier versions of your favorite foods.

Habits to Adopt

- Slowly take out things from your diet one at a time.
- Hold a family meeting to gain and gauge your family's support for sticking to a nutrient-dense, low-carbohydrate menu.
- Host a taste test of non-wheat pastas to find out which ones you like.
- Give up refined carbohydrates for one full day (just to try it and see).
- Keep a food journal for a week to watch when cravings for carbohydrate-loaded and processed foods strike.
- Purchase a meal subscription that focuses on low-carbohydrate meals.
- Try low-carb or no-carb alternatives to satisfy your pasta cravings.
- Put any processed/snack foods in a locked cabinet in the basement or attic.
- Fill two-thirds of your plate with vegetables and nutrient-dense foods at every meal.
- Plan your snacks ahead of time with pre-portioned amounts of nuts, vegetables, and other low-carbohydrate snacks.
- Brush your teeth immediately after dinner each day.

- Replace your rice and pasta with low-carb or no-carb options like cauliflower rice and shirataki noodles.

- Eliminate packaged and processed foods that contain trans fats and high sodium: boxed cake mixes, store-bought cookies and pastries, microwavable frozen meals, foods listing "hydrogenated" or "partially hydrogenated oils" on the ingredients list, like vegetable shortening and margarine.

- Reduce your consumption of saturated fats (from animal meat and dairy). This is due to a suboptimal APOA2 gene.

- Prioritize polyunsaturated fats (fats from plants), especially omega-3 fatty acids. Marine sources: algae, wild fatty fish such as anchovies, mackerel, sardines, salmon, and cod; plant sources of omega 3s: avocado oil, flaxseed oil, walnuts, flaxseeds, chia seeds, hemp seeds, edamame, seaweed.

- When shopping, buy the low- or no-fat version of dairy products like yogurt and milk.

- Wash and package vegetables for easy snacking when you go to your refrigerator.

- Institute (or expand) a "meatless Monday" plan for yourself or your family when you focus on replacing high-fat dairy or meat with vegetable alternatives like tofu, butternut squash, jackfruit, or beets.

- Dedicate at least one day per week to perfecting a stir-fry or roasted vegetable recipe that you enjoy.

- Buy an easy-to-eat option from the list of omega-3-rich items: smoked salmon, sardines, roasted seaweed, guacamole (with flaxseed chips), etc.

- Buy a book with microbiome-friendly recipes.

- Rid your pantry and medicine cabinet of any toiletries or foods with preservatives, food colorings, and artificial sweeteners.

- Talk to your doctor about reducing medications, if possible. If pregnant, discuss the benefits of vaginal birth.

- Read up on the negative effects of antibiotics and understand their optimal (not reactive) use.

- Purchase and taste test an array of fermented foods you don't regularly buy: kefir, krauts, kombucha, kimchi, etc.

- Reduce any exposure to chemicals and pesticides in products ranging from cleaning products to toiletries, allowing exposure to healthy, natural environments.

- Eat favorite prebiotics twice daily: chocolate with high percentage cacao, artichoke hearts, bananas, etc.

- Walk in the dirt or grass barefoot for a few minutes each day.

- Eat one type of fermented food each morning with your breakfast.

Behaviors to Avoid

- Overdoing it on a select few types of low-carb foods— you'll quickly become bored of it and you'll end up going back to carbs.

- Going strong on a high-fat diet—review your profile with a health care practitioner before jumping into any diet!

- Eating as much beans, chickpeas, and quinoa as you like—these are all still sources of carbs, and the high amounts of fiber over time can actually contribute to stomach problems if you don't prepare them properly or you eat them excessively.

- Overdoing it on plant fats like avocados, olive oil, nuts, and seeds.

- Choosing low-fat food products that are high in sodium instead to make up for the lack of fat and flavor.

- Completely ignoring fats in your diet—some fats are still important to a healthy diet!

- Eating processed foods—replace them with a variety of natural, fresh foods.

- Eating foods that are dried from chemicals such as chickpeas.
- Storing and heating food in plastic containers.
- Going overboard with "cleanliness"—constantly using hand sanitizer and mouthwash can destroy healthy bacteria and actually make you more susceptible to sickness due to a weakened immune system.

Supplements

- Blood Sugar Optimizer
- Berberine
- Alpha-lipoic acid

Finally, one more reminder: the genomic recommendations listed above were intended to provide *me* with guidance on how to mitigate the impact of various health outcomes that could influence *my* overall diet and nutrition profile. I relate more to some health concerns than others. But *you* need to talk to *your* doctor about how you can implement the recommendations you receive in a safe and supervised manner.

Chapter 6

·•∴•∴•∴•∴•∴•∴•

DNA AND SLEEP

*The way to a more productive, more inspired,
more joyful life is getting enough sleep.*

— ARIANNA HUFFINGTON, AUTHOR, COLUMNIST,
AND FOUNDER AND CEO OF THRIVE GLOBAL

The fastest recorded smash of a Ping-Pong ball is 70 miles per hour, which New Zealander Lark Brandt achieved at the World's Fastest Smash Competition in 2003. Impressive, but did you know it's possible for a Ping-Pong ball, under the right circumstances, to travel 2,484 miles per hour? At that speed, about Mach 3 and 3,694 feet per second—faster than an F-16 fighter jet—the humble Ping-Pong ball can fly faster than the speed of sound.

No wonder Ping-Pong players stand so far back from the table.

Now, take 1,000 starving and poor Ping-Pong players, cram them into a tiny room, tell them they can win an Olympic gold medal if they just want it bad enough, and have them smash shots that break the sound barrier until there's one person left standing.

That's what it's like inside my head when I'm trying to go to sleep. And that's why, when I began my health journey, I was advised to look at how I sleep.

Getting a good night's sleep has always been a challenge for me. Growing up in a cramped apartment, often going to sleep hungry, and planning a big future for myself when I was supposed to be sleeping didn't help.

As an adult, and especially as an entrepreneur, the speed and frenetic activity of my life can be hard to manage. On one shoulder, an anxious and ambitious guy—call him Kashif One—says, "How can you sleep when there's so much to do!?" On the other shoulder, a nagging but well-meaning guy—call him Kashif Two—says, "You know that if you want to prevent and reverse illness, live longer, and perform at your best, getting a good night's sleep is as vital as diet and exercise."

"Tell that to my investors," says Kashif One.

"But Kashif One," says Kashif Two, "if you don't go to sleep, you'll be in a bad mood, your brain won't work like it should, and your health will suffer."

To which Kashif One replies, "Sleep, schmeep. I've got deals to close. Products to launch. I'm changing health care!"

Kashif Two sighs and says, "Not getting enough quality sleep raises the risks of heart disease, stroke, obesity, dementia, and other disorders. You know this."

On and on it goes, with heaping doses of esoteric information and ephemera, like how fast a Ping-Pong ball can travel, cluttering my mind for hours and not letting me go to sleep.

After looking at my genomic test results and listening to my team of researchers and clinicians, I realized the number of hours I was spending in bed wasn't the issue, although I could've done better in that category. The more important questions were: How much sleep was I getting? Was I consistently getting that sleep? Was my sleep of high quality, meaning, did I sleep without waking, and did I feel renewed in the morning?

The answer was no on all counts. And I'm not alone.

According to the CDC, sleep disorders are so pervasive in the United States—again, I'm using the U.S. as a stand-in for Western society—they now constitute a public health epidemic that manifests in several ways. For instance, research conducted by the CDC indicates that nearly 50 million Americans admit to having problems concentrating during the day due to lack of sleep, 24 million people admit they don't drive as well, and 18 million people admit their job performance has suffered.

Notice I said Americans "admit" before those statistics. That's because our society seems to think being sleepy is weak and something to be ashamed of. We're supposed to "push through" the fatigue, pull "all-nighters" to get the job done, and "grind it out" no matter what. We take pride in our "go-go-go hustle culture" and scoff at those who don't.

For instance, I read somewhere that Lou Gerstner, Jr., the former CEO of IBM, said he knew IBM would come back from the brink of bankruptcy in the '90s when at the end of his workday—sometime after midnight—he saw most of the lights on in the building and the parking lot still filled with employees' cars. That was a clear message to employees: if you care enough about the company, and you want to personally succeed and be lionized for your efforts, you will ignore your biological needs at all costs. Although IBM did have one of the most impressive turnarounds in business history, the load being put on its employees was insane and unsustainable. But this attitude was so valued in the company that I also know people used to purposely leave their office lights on and their cars in the parking lot—someone would pick them up because they were too tired to drive—because they wanted to make it *seem* like they were still working.

I'm not telling this story to slam IBM. I'm telling it because IBM is emblematic of America's larger culture of work. And if you think you would never succumb to the pressure of working like those IBM employees did, think again. Think of all the times you or someone you know have fallen asleep while watching TV or a movie or attending one of your kids' school plays, and upon being awakened by an elbow to the ribs, you said, "I wasn't sleeping!" We've all been there.

In addition to having trouble concentrating, driving, and working, sleep disorders such as insomnia and obstructive sleep apnea are placing those who suffer from these conditions and the public-at-large at greater risk of car crashes, medical mistakes, and industrial accidents. Moreover, sleep disorders represent an increasing risk to public health, contributing to a host of medical conditions, including cancer, obesity, diabetes, depression, and hypertension.

And that's before we even talk about teens.

According to a 2006 National Sleep Foundation poll, by their senior year, only about 15 percent of high school students get enough quality sleep. The average high school student gets only 6.5 hours of sleep a night, when they should be getting at least 9; and 20 percent of teens sleep 5 or fewer hours a night. This all adds up to a serious threat to teens' health, safety, and academic success. Sleep deprivation increases the likelihood teens will suffer myriad negative consequences, including an inability to concentrate, poor grades, drowsy-driving incidents, anxiety, depression, thoughts of suicide, and even suicide attempts. This is regardless of socioeconomic status.

As a result, we are setting up teens for a lifetime of illness, shorter life expectancies, and poor performance when we should be setting them up for success with better sleep habits.

So why do we need to sleep anyway?

People think of sleep as "resting," when their exhausted brain gets a break. But your brain performs many important functions when it's asleep. For instance, when you're sleeping, your brain acts like a purification system that flushes out toxins and prepares to learn, remember, and create. Every system in your body repairs itself while you sleep. If you don't get enough sleep, your systems will not be able to handle the strain put upon them.

How much sleep do you need? Experts say elementary school children and middle schoolers should get at least 9 hours a night and teens should get between 8 and 10. Most adults need at least 7 hours or more of sleep each night.

Okay, you say. But if you work around the clock on a big project for a couple of weeks, you can catch up on sleep when the project is over, right? No, you can't. If you occasionally have a late night, you can take a nap the next day or sleep longer and maybe feel better. But there is no way you can recover from being chronically sleep deprived.

On the other hand, sleeping too much is also a problem. If you're sleeping for 10 or 12 hours every night and waking up groggy, there might be something else going on, like a sleep disorder such as insomnia, where you can't get to sleep and have trouble staying asleep. Another common sleep disorder is sleep apnea, where your upper airway becomes blocked and you stop breathing. Constantly waking up several times a minute means you never get into a place of restorative sleep.

If you're having trouble sleeping, you should get tested at a sleep disorder clinic. I know someone who got tested after years of snoring like a lawnmower and getting repeatedly nudged by his wife to switch positions. The clinician recorded the test on video because clients often don't believe they're snoring and seeing the video helps to convince them. In my friend's case, they stopped the session after five minutes because he had one of the worst cases of sleep apnea they had ever seen. When they showed him the video what he saw was scary. He was gasping and sputtering, choking like someone had their hands around his neck, and not breathing at all for 10 seconds at a time. They advised him to try sleeping that night in the clinic in a CPAP mask that provides a continuous flow of oxygen to keep the upper airway open. They would observe him and record him and see how he felt in the morning. He agreed. When he woke up, he felt so refreshed and alert he said it was as if he'd never slept before. He didn't need to look at the video because he felt it. He was clearheaded and full of energy.

If that story doesn't tell you how important getting quality sleep is, I don't know what will. The clinician made my friend's life better in every way, and may have even saved it.

So what do your genes have to do with sleep?

Your genes play an important role in achieving, maintaining, and benefiting from quality sleep by influencing your response to factors such as food, lifestyle, and the environment. When you get your DNA tested you receive a report that looks at a number of these important genes and how variations in them can increase or decrease your likelihood of achieving restful and beneficial sleep.

Here are my test results.

Gene Tested	COMT	DRD2	ADR-A2B	5-HT-TLPR	MAO	CLOCK	BDNF	SOD2
Result	GG	AA	ID	SS	GG	TT	GG	CC

Gene Tested	CY-P2R1	VDBP/GC	FTO	MC4R	VDR	GSTT1	GSTM1	GSTP1	GPX
Result	AG	CC	TT	CT	CT	1	0	AA	CC

Next, I'll tell you what that means across five key areas impacting quality of sleep: circadian rhythms, stress, pleasure, environment, and food.

Circadian Rhythms

Circadian rhythms are 24-hour cycles that are part of the body's internal clock, running in the background to carry out essential biological processes that occur throughout the day, from when you wake up until you fall asleep. Levels of certain hormones such as melatonin, testosterone, and cortisol are all influenced by your sleep-wake cycle. As the day transitions into night, darkness prompts your body to release melatonin and start to lower its temperature. Melatonin levels are highest in the evening into the later parts of the night. Cortisol levels peak during the day, while testosterone levels are highest in the early hours of the morning and between 5 and 7 in the evening.

One of the most important and well-known circadian rhythms is the sleep-wake cycle, which can be influenced by genetic variations. For example, weak genetic variations might cause your sleep-wake cycle to be disrupted, making it harder for you to fall asleep, stay asleep, or achieve deep, restful sleep so you wake up feeling refreshed.

In my case, the genes that influence my circadian rhythms are not optimal. This means, based on my genetics, I am more likely to have irregular or disrupted circadian rhythms when it comes to my sleep. On top of that, the choices I make complicate matters that much more.

For example, I'm writing these words at 5 A.M., which is not the best time for a night owl like me. But my schedule last night and this morning has dictated when I could make time to write today. So, this is what I've chosen.

I tell you this because when we make trade-offs that sacrifice sleep, like I'm doing, whether it's through pounding pots of coffee or sheer force of will, we can probably perform tasks that are out of our normal rhythms. Like writing. Normally I'd be doing this at 9 or 10 in the evening. That happens to be the best time for me to write. Other people are different. My co-author, for instance, is a morning person and playwright who used to get up at 4 in the morning and drink a lot of coffee so he could write plays before his *normal* work-day started. That was probably too early, even for a morning person, and he'll be the first to tell you that his health took a hit because of it. He doesn't do that anymore, not because he's stopped writing plays (he hasn't), but because he's prioritizing his health. I don't drink coffee, so I bulldoze my way through fatigue, which is also not helpful. I try to counteract that by taking naps. But the bottom line is this: whichever way you fight your own sleep-regulation processes, your health is going to suffer.

When you make the trade-off I've described above, and you chronically ignore or override the circadian rhythm that regulates your sleep-wake cycle, you create chaos in everything from hormone levels and cellular processes to body temperature and brain waves. As a result of this misalignment, you get conditions like brain fog, cancer, and metabolic syndrome (high blood pressure, high blood sugar, elevated cholesterol, and excess waistline fat that can raise the risk for heart disease, type 2 diabetes, and stroke).

If you understand your genetics, you can make more informed choices about how you interact with your circadian rhythms.

Let's take a closer look at my genome.

The CLOCK gene is thought to play an important role in controlling circadian rhythms, particularly the sleep-wake cycle. Variations in this gene influence the body's ability to fall asleep and the risk of mood-related disorders, as well as the response to certain kinds of diets in persons of some ethnicities (Chinese), and the risk of obesity. The TT genotype is associated with normal sleep patterns, while the CT and CC genotypes result in delayed and irregular sleep function as well as an increased risk of insomnia, depression, bipolar disorder, and other mood-related behavioral disorders.

My CLOCK genotype is TT, which is the optimal version of the gene. That means I am more likely to have normal sleep-wake circadian rhythms.

BDNF, found in areas of the brain that control eating, sleeping, and overall mood balance, is an important neurochemical involved in neural plasticity. In other words, it controls the efficiency with which your neurons (brain cells) can form new connections. BDNF influences the health, growth, and maintenance of your neurons (the cells found in your brain and nervous system). Low levels of BDNF have been linked to an increased risk of insomnia and other mood-related disorders.

Variations within your BDNF gene can influence the levels of BDNF in the brain. As it relates to sleep, studies have shown that individuals with lower levels of BDNF are more likely to struggle with achieving rested sleep, even after longer periods (seven to eight hours). They are also more likely to display symptoms of insomnia and are more likely to struggle with changes in time zones and jet lag. Furthermore, studies have shown that individuals with low BDNF are more likely to be influenced negatively by digital screen time prior to bed.

My BDNF genotype is GG, which is the optimal version.

Your vitamin D genes play an important role in your ability to absorb, transport, and activate vitamin D.

My VDBP/GC genotype is CC, which is the optimal version. This means I efficiently transport vitamin D in my body from the site of activation to the site of action.

However, because I carry the suboptimal version of the CYP2R1 gene (AG), I don't effectively convert vitamin D_2 from the sun (ergocalciferol) into activated vitamin D_3 (cholecalciferol).

Finally, your VDR gene controls the efficiency with which vitamin D binds to its receptor and activates its effect on your cells. My

VDR genotype is CT, which is suboptimal. This version is linked to poor vitamin D binding and activation at the receptor site.

Vitamin D is one of the most important hormones in the body, and part of its function lies in regulating sleep cycles. Studies have linked lower levels of vitamin D to a higher risk of disturbed sleep, poor-quality sleep, and a reduced duration of sleep.

If you get tested and find you have suboptimal variations of these genes, you are more likely to be affected by factors that disrupt your sleep, such as stress, jet lag, shift work, screen time, stimulants and depressants, exercise, and even your diet.

Bedtime Battlefield

Sometimes when we talk to clients who are having trouble sleeping, they describe feeling like they're under attack. In a sense they are, tossing and turning in bed for hours on end fighting their "attackers"—stress from a situation, the environment in which they're living, the food they ate that didn't agree with them, or their own addictive tendencies.

We can tell them how important sleep is, but that doesn't make it any easier. In some cases, it makes it worse, because they know they need to sleep, but they can't seem to make it happen. However, while we can't necessarily remove their attackers, we can help them defend themselves based on their genetics.

Our genes play an important role in our ability to achieve, maintain, and benefit from optimal sleep by influencing our response to factors such as food, lifestyle, and the environment. When we test a client's genome and prepare a report, we look at a number of these important genes, specifically how variations in these genes can increase or decrease our predisposition toward optimal sleep outcomes.

As always, it's important to remember that functional genomics requires the understanding that genes are only part of the overall construction. Your predisposition toward suboptimal or poor outcomes is not diagnostic and does not necessarily mean you *will* suffer from the associated outcomes. Similarly, an optimal genetic profile does not guarantee that you will not suffer from poor sleep length or quality. A comprehensive review of your dietary, lifestyle, and environmental choices is necessary to build a complete picture of the factors that could be affecting your sleep. Our goal with any client is to personalize and help you find the solutions needed to achieve optimal sleep.

Let's look at a few of the attackers you might face when trying to sleep, and the genes associated with them. As before, I'll share my own genetic results.

Stress

Stress is a biological response to the changes you experience throughout your life. It is your body's safety and defense mechanism. Our ancient ancestors felt it when they were on the run from a saber-toothed tiger, and it protected them. But today, we still feel the same response even if it's something that's comparatively slight, such as an argument with a friend, family member, or co-worker. However, an inability to appropriately address and manage the daily stressors in your life may lead to chronic stress, typically accompanied by chronic poor sleep. Which lead to attacks on our biological functions.

As noted earlier, there are many biological functions that occur during sleep, and not all at the same time. Dreaming, for example, occurs during rapid eye movement (REM) sleep. Up to 75 percent of our sleep is considered non-REM sleep, while approximately 25 percent is considered REM sleep. REM sleep cycles occur in approximately 90-minute cycles. However, it's during deep sleep that our bodies enter a rested state where many critical rest and recovery processes take place. Waking up during deep sleep can cause excessive fatigue, grogginess, or drowsiness since our body must come out of a deeper stage of sleep. If stress is getting to you while you're trying to fall asleep or stay asleep, it's going to hurt you.

Taken together, the genes that influence how I handle stress are suboptimal. This means stress is likely to play an influential role in the quality of my sleep based on my genetics.

Your COMT gene influences the efficiency of your COMT enzyme, which is involved in the metabolism and clearance of important neurotransmitters like dopamine and noradrenaline. Individuals with a slow COMT AA genotype are more likely to be influenced by stress and stay stressed for longer periods of time than others.

My COMT GG genotype is the fast version, which is not commonly associated with an increased or heightened stress response.

Your ADRA2B gene controls your noradrenaline receptor. A partial "ID" or full deletion DD in this gene can cause your receptor to stay "on" for a longer period, which allows noradrenaline to bind to it and keep you in a heightened emotional state that is often associated with stress and anxiety. If you also carry the slow COMT gene (I do not), which takes a longer time to metabolize noradrenaline, then your risk of being significantly influenced by stress and anxiety increases as well.

My ADRA2B ID genotype is suboptimal. This means I am more likely to be impacted by the emotional events I experience and more likely to let my emotions drive my response.

Stressful situations can cause me to stay up all night worrying about them. My genetic test results indicate that I may replay negative events in my mind and have a harder time letting go of things.

Your SLC6A4 gene is your serotonin transport gene. A polymorphism within this gene known as 5-HTTLPR can influence the efficiency of your serotonin pathway. Individuals with a "short" or "S" version in one or both alleles of this polymorphism experience dysregulated serotonin uptake. This can influence their ability to recognize and address emotional stimuli in an appropriate manner. These individuals tend to display a lower threshold for irritation and are more likely to become visibly frustrated or distracted by emotional stimuli than others.

My 5-HTTLPR SS genotype is suboptimal. This means I am more likely to have a dysregulated serotonin response.

Serotonin plays an important role in sleep and circadian rhythm management. When your serotonin is dysregulated, you can find it harder to fall or stay asleep particularly when you're stressed. You're also more likely to become stressed about things far quicker than others are.

Pleasure

The feeling of pleasure is one that most people commonly associate with happiness and positivity. However, your pursuit of pleasure may lead to addiction. Whether you can't get enough of that good feeling or can't let go of that good feeling, addiction (and, by extension, depression and anxiety resulting from the addiction) can hinder the ability to develop a healthy sleep cycle.

Like my stress profile, the genes that influence how I handle pleasure are suboptimal. This means pleasure will have a negative impact on my ability to get quality sleep.

Variations in your genes can influence how long and how much pleasure you experience. This can influence your mood, behavior, and daily habits—which in turn can impact your ability to fall asleep, stay asleep, or keep a regular sleep schedule.

I carry the fast COMT GG and MAO GG genotypes. This may affect my sleep cycle because those genotypes mean I am more likely to have an increased risk of displaying addictive and depressive tendencies, particularly when I feel unfulfilled by my lifestyle or career, for example.

My low DRD2 AA genotype decreases my ability to feel emotions like pleasure and anxiety. Practically speaking, I'm likely to schedule my days around accomplishing goals or around the things that bring me pleasure. As a result, my desire to engage in pleasurable tasks may influence my ability to prepare for or fall asleep.

Environment

The different environments in your daily life profoundly impact your health and wellness, including the length and quality of your sleep. Important gene variations in your DNA influence your ability to process environmental agents that enter your body. This processing occurs during sleep, so poor sleep can significantly hamper your ability to deal with these toxins. The better you manage these environmental agents, the more likely you are to have a healthy detoxification profile, which contributes to optimal sleep quality.

As in the case with stress and pleasure, I have a suboptimal profile when it comes to the genes that influence my response to my environment. Because I have a suboptimal detoxification profile, environmental agents like those found in pollution, smog, cigarette smoke, mold, perfumes, and household chemicals wreak havoc on my body by causing cellular inflammation. Cellular inflammation is one of the hallmarks of chronic disease. Individuals with poor detoxification profiles often suffer with migraines, chronic fatigue, and lack of energy, along with a host of other health concerns. I discussed this earlier in regard to the toxins in our new office and how I responded to them—not well.

These health concerns impact sleep quality because they disrupt our ability to fall asleep, feel rested, and complete daily tasks without difficulty. They also leave us feeling uncomfortable and stressed out, which can prevent us from falling asleep at the proper time.

GSTT1, GSTM1 and GSTP1

Your GST family of enzymes controls the efficiency of your glutathione pathway. Glutathione is the most important detox pathway in your body and is responsible for the metabolism and clearance of many environmental toxins. Variations in your GST family of genes influence the efficiency of their respective enzymes. The GSTT1 gene influences the efficiency of the GSTT1 enzyme and is generally responsible for the removal of free radicals or oxidants, which can cause mitochondrial and overall cellular damage. This is often displayed as fatigue, tiredness, and lack of energy. The GSTP1 gene influences the efficiency of the GSTP1 enzyme, which is involved in the removal of toxins like mold, cigarette smoke, perfumes, and polyaromatic hydrocarbons. Outcomes of a poor GSTP1 result often include migraines, nerve pain, and muscle pain.

With one copy of the GSTT1 gene, I have an average ability to remove toxins and harmful agents from my body.

However, I am missing both copies of the GSTM1 gene—I do not have this gene in my DNA. As a result, my ability to remove toxins and other harmful substances is significantly reduced. Because of that, I am more likely to recover slowly and experience greater symptoms of fatigue, being overly tired, or lacking energy. All true.

All is not lost, however, because I also carry the optimal version of the GSTP1 gene. This means I am more likely to manage and remove heavy metals from my body, as well as resist sensory overload when it comes to strong smells and scents.

SOD2 and GPX

Your SOD2 and GPX enzymes play an important role in the removal of oxidants. Oxidants can damage your mitochondria, which are the power plants of your cells, where the production of energy occurs. A slower SOD2 enzyme, resulting from variations in your SOD2 gene, can result in the buildup of oxidants in your cells. This may result in outcomes such as fatigue and lack of energy. A slower GPX enzyme doesn't convert hydrogen peroxide, which is formed by SOD2, into water and oxygen as quickly. This can result in a buildup of hydrogen peroxide in your cells, which can be harmful to your health.

In my case, I convert harmful, fatigue-causing oxidants into hydrogen peroxide at an increased rate via the superoxide dismutase (SOD2) pathway. I also convert hydrogen peroxide into water and diatomic oxygen at an increased rate. When it comes to SOD2 and GPX, I'm a healthy little conversion factory.

Note: If you get your genome tested and find you also have the TT version of the SOD2 gene, you may want to speak to your practitioner about monitoring your hydrogen peroxide levels to ensure you're maintaining appropriate levels.

Food

Your diet plays an incredibly important role in your sleep schedule. This includes what, how, and when you eat. Your genes control several dietary functions involved in your ability to break down certain macronutrients like fats and carbohydrates. They also influence your ability to feel full, when you get hunger cravings, and how you respond to certain foods like salty, sugary, or fried foods. These functions can influence your ability to get a good night's rest.

I have a suboptimal profile when it comes to the genes that influence my relationship with food. Because of this, my genetic relationship with food is more likely to have a negative impact on the quality of my sleep.

Your FTO gene influences your satiety response. Satiety refers to your ability to feel full after consuming food. When you eat a meal, your body monitors the food being consumed and sends a signal to your brain once it believes you've reached your capacity. However, for some people, variations in their genes can cause these signals to become disrupted, making it harder for them to realize when they are full and when they are hungry. As a result, they tend to overestimate their ability to eat and often overeat during meals. They are also more likely to go hunting for a snack, particularly later at night. Eating at night and overeating both contribute to dysregulated sleep cycles because the body is forced to perform digestive duties during a time when it should be focused on rest and recovery. Eating at night pushes the circadian rhythm back further, making it difficult to fall asleep until much later. That's why, regardless of genetics, we should aim to stop eating at least two or three hours before going to bed.

Luckily for me, I have the optimal version of the FTO gene, which means, based on my genetics, I should have normal satiety and eating behaviors.

Your MC4R gene controls your hunger cues by controlling the feedback loop between your stomach and your mind. Like the FTO gene, variations in the MC4R gene can inhibit that feedback loop, which can cause dysregulated snacking patterns. Individuals with the C allele are more likely to hunt for snacks or graze throughout the day, particularly at night and particularly when they are not stimulated. They are also more likely to overeat if their snack is not variable enough to provide different sensory profiles to the mouth, such as the sensation of sweet, salty, crunchy, crispy, bitter, sour, or fatty. If you have a snacking tendency, make sure your snack is built with protein and healthy fats, not just carbs like chips, crackers, bread, etc.

In my case, I have a suboptimal version of the MC4R gene. This means I have dysregulated hunger cues. As a result, I'm more likely to engage in snacking or grazing behaviors throughout the day and into the night, which may influence my ability to fall asleep at the right time.

Due to a suboptimal AMY1 genotype, I carry an increased association between a diet high in starches and weight gain. This may contribute to metabolic dysfunction at night when my body is trying to sleep and repair itself.

Finally, due to a suboptimal TCF7L2 genotype (insulin sensitivity) there is an increased likelihood that I'll develop hyperglycemia (elevated blood sugar) if I eat a diet high in starches. This means I should avoid eating processed or added sugars in general and moderate my fruit consumption. I should also keep fruit consumption during the day to avoid glucose spikes at night, which contribute to metabolic dysfunction.

If you think it's hard getting yourself to sleep, try getting a toddler to do it.

That's the story behind Adam Mansbach's *New York Times* best-selling book *Go the Fuck to Sleep.* Tired and testy, Mansbach was enduring yet another four-hour battle to get his three-year-old daughter to sleep when he joked on social media that he was going to write a book with that name. Many of his friends, most of whom had experienced the same difficulty with their children, saw the post and encouraged him to follow through and write the book.

As of 2019, the book has been translated into 40 languages and sold more than 3 million copies. This profane children's book for adults is popular because so many adults, me included, can easily identify with it.

Also, how many times have you laid awake in bed, tormented by insomnia over something—the meatball and onion sandwich you ate too late, the still-floating toxins from the yard work done by a neighbor earlier that day, the just-one-more game you love playing on your smartphone—and said those words to yourself? I know I have.

After I got my DNA tested and analyzed, my team recommended some sleep-specific actions I could take based on my genome. I share them with you now to show you what helps me sleep better, given my genetics, lifestyle, diet and nutrition, and environment.

While some people may have a genetic profile similar to mine, I have no idea if these recommendations would work for you—and neither do you unless you get tested. So please understand these recommendations are for me. You have to get your own!

Circadian Rhythms

Lifestyle

- Build a consistent sleep schedule using proper sleep hygiene (blackout curtains, lower room temperature, cold pillows, aromatherapy, comfortable clothing, no screens in the bed).
- Ensure adequate exposure to sunlight throughout the year and every morning to start your clock.
- Build a regular exercise schedule with low intensity in the evening and high intensity during the day.

Habits to Adopt

- Buy a noise machine and an essential oil diffuser for your bedroom and use both every night to get you ready for sleep.
- Go outside every morning after breakfast for a vigorous 5- to 10-minute walk.
- Open all the blinds in your home to increase daylight exposure.
- Turn your phone on Do Not Disturb mode after 5 P.M.
- Stop eating a few hours before bed to allow for vibrant metabolic health.
- Swap your cup of coffee for a cup of yerba mate, which contains a cousin of caffeine known as mateine that provides a longer-lasting energy boost without as much of a crash as caffeine.

Behaviors to Avoid

- Stimulants like caffeine, alcohol, or recreational substances at night.
- Excessive phone or digital screen time, particularly at night.
- Long naps during the day, which can increase your risk of disrupted sleep-wake cycles.

Supplements

- BDNF Optimizer
- Vitamin D

Stress

Lifestyle

- Avoid toxic relationships—address the situation with the individual or make a conscious decision to move on from that relationship.
- Engage in tasks that make you happy directly after a stressful situation to improve your overall mood and response.

Habits to Adopt

- Keep a daily log of all the things that cause you stress, then write down whether you can actively do something about addressing them, one at a time.
- As the shower warms up, practice one form of mindfulness for 30 to 60 seconds.
- After you notice anything pleasant, stand quietly and take a moment to ground yourself in the present moment.
- Take a walk outside and name what you see aloud: a bird, a type of tree, clouds, etc. Marvel in the beauty of the simple things.
- Pause momentarily for a quiet moment of gratitude at the start of a meal.

- As you wait in the checkout line, do a deep-breathing exercise.

Behaviors to Avoid

- Worrying about things from your past.
- Worrying excessively about the future.
- Overworking yourself to the point of exhaustion.

Supplements

- Ashwagandha
- L-theanine
- Rhodiola
- Ginseng
- Deep Calm Optimizer
- Sleep Optimizer

Pleasure

Lifestyle

- Research how a beginner gets started learning an activity you might enjoy. YouTube is a great source for such things.
- Seek out a club or group that regularly does the pleasure activity you seek, like reading books, skiing, or cooking.
- Purchase supplies for the new pleasure activities that will help you get started.
- Hire a personal coach to help you level up your skills quickly.
- Remove all the addictive pleasure activity paraphernalia from your home: ashtrays, vaporizers, video consoles, etc.

Habits to Adopt

- Do your recreational pleasure activity at the same time each day/week.

- Include your partner/friend in sharing the results or what you make.
- Write a blog or Instagram post about each milestone you reach.
- Give away extra materials or completed books to people in need once you're done with each project.
- Make a place in your home to take time for the pleasure activity.

Behaviors to Avoid

- Engaging in behaviors that "feel" good but aren't necessarily good for your mental and physical health.
- Waiting until you are exhausted at the end of the day to do something you enjoy.
- Falling back into repetitive habits at the first sign of resistance—remember that change is hard, but the outcome is worth it!

Environment

Lifestyle

- Purchase an air-purifying plant for each room of your home.
- Clear your home of toxic cleaning products and toiletries.
- Learn about green cleaning chemicals and techniques.
- Dispose of all the plastic products in your household.
- Purchase a set of glassware containers for food storage.

Habits to Adopt

- Purchase cleaning products and toiletries that are packaged in glass bottles.
- Vacuum each day after the final meal.
- Replace your air filter once every three months.

- Clean one room of your home after breakfast.
- Open the windows upon waking to allow fresh air to circulate.
- Dust your home on the weekend.
- Turn on an air purifier each morning.

Behaviors to Avoid

- Using harsh chemicals in cleaning products.
- Wearing shoes inside your home.
- Using synthetic fragrances and air fresheners.

Food

Diet

- Focus on nutritionally dense meals that help you feel full—speak to a nutritionist or health coach to build a plan based on your diet and nutrition profile.
- Avoid foods with "empty calories"—these are foods high in sugars or starchy carbohydrates that can often induce overeating or grazing behavior.

Lifestyle

- Buy ingredients for effective and fulfilling snacks.
- Sign an agreement with your family that you won't use devices when eating a meal or at the table.
- Attend a class or seminar on mindful eating.
- Talk to your doctor about intermittent fasting two times a week.
- Subscribe to a podcast on mindful eating habits.

Habits to Adopt

- Put your fork down between bites.
- Slow down your chewing between bites.
- Always have a nutritious snack on hand that meets specific criteria.

- Clean produce upon arriving home from the store.
- Do food prep each weekend to ensure you have nutritious foods on hand.

Behaviors to Avoid

- Screen use during mealtime.
- Eating frequently at all-you-can-eat venues or buffet restaurants.
- Eating pre-packaged or instant meals out of boxes.
- Eating less than two hours before bed.

Remember, optimal sleep quality is about more than just sleeping at the right time. When you approach the goal of improving your sleep in a functional manner by looking at the various ways your genes can impact your sleep, you are more likely to succeed in the long run. As always, you should review your plans with your clinical provider prior to implementing any recommendations with regards to your health and wellness.

Chapter 7

DNA AND CARDIOVASCULAR HEALTH

If you are over the age of 10, the question isn't whether or not to eat healthy to prevent heart disease. It's whether or not you want to reverse the heart disease you already have.

— MICHAEL GREGER, M.D., PUBLIC HEALTH EXPERT AND *NEW YORK TIMES* BEST-SELLING AUTHOR OF *HOW NOT TO DIE*

According to the CDC, heart disease is currently the leading cause of death both in the U.S. and worldwide. On average, someone dies from cardiovascular disease every 34 seconds, which is around 2,541 deaths per day.

I should point out here that the term *heart disease* describes several different conditions, many of which relate to the buildup of plaque in a person's arteries or irregular heart rhythms.

This topic goes straight to my heart.

Earlier, I talked about my own father dying of an unexpected but preventable heart attack when I was 17 years old, and how that devastated my family and changed my life. I also talked about how one of my closest friends was dealing with cardiovascular issues and getting no help for it until my colleagues at The DNA Company stepped in. And I can't tell you how many clients we've worked with—such as the NHL hockey player I spoke of earlier and thousands of other people—to help them address their heart-related challenges; it's rewarding to see their improvements and know we had something to do with making that happen.

Let's talk about how we do that.

The DNA Company's approach to cardiovascular health is based on understanding the steps involved in chronic inflammation. We evaluate a few important factors to give you a thorough picture of your cardiovascular profile.

We ask how inflammation occurs in the body. What is the impact of inflammatory toxins in the bloodstream? How quickly are these toxins metabolized and removed from the bloodstream? How efficient is the body's response to these toxins?

Toxins enter your bloodstream through both internal processes (such as free radicals or estrogen metabolites) and external factors (such as sugar, simple carbohydrates, mold, smoke, pollution, chemicals, etc.). These toxins make their way into your bloodstream where, if they stay around long enough, they can initiate an inflammatory response along the endothelial (inner) lining of your blood vessels. The efficiency with which your body can remove these toxins is influenced by several functional genes.

If your ability to remove these toxins is not as great as it should be, then the tolerance of your blood vessels toward toxins comes into play. How protective or resistant to inflammation your blood vessels are is significantly influenced by variations found in your DNA. Some individuals have "Teflon-coated" or "bulletproof" blood vessels that can resist significantly higher levels of toxins in the bloodstream than normal. Other individuals have blood vessels that are more susceptible to toxins in the bloodstream and thus are more likely to become inflamed in the presence of these toxins.

If the body has a lower tolerance to these toxins, then inflammation starts to occur. The efficiency of your cellular anti-inflammatory response, driven by a cellular cycle known as methylation, determines how quickly you can address the inflammation where it occurs. In addition to this process, the body also releases cholesterol when inflammation occurs.

Cholesterol is an important molecule in our body that acts as an anti-inflammatory agent at the site of inflammation. Think of it as the body's internal lubricant. How well your body moves cholesterol to and from the site of inflammation influences whether cholesterol will harden at the site of inflammation and cause the buildup of plaque. This will ultimately influence your risk of high cholesterol.

In this section, I will explore the various genes and internal processes that influence your individual response and predisposition to the processes we mentioned above.

I will also evaluate three important health concerns that contribute to your overall likelihood of developing cardiovascular disease, as well as share some clinical recommendations I received to improve my diet and lifestyle and reduce my overall likelihood of cardiovascular disease.

Here are my own test results:

Gene Tested	MTR	MTRR	SHMT1	MTHFR	9P21	IP21
Result	AG	GG	GG	CC	3G	AG

Gene Tested	APOE3	ACE	FUT2	NOS3	AMY1	SOD2	PCSK9
Result	3/3	AA	GG	GG	AA	CC	GG

Gene Tested	SLCO1B1	APOA2	TCF7L2	GSTT1 (copies)	GSTM1 (copies)	GSTP1	GPX
Result	TT	GG	TT	1	0	AA	CC

I realize this must look like a complicated table for an eye test. In the next section, I'll tell you what these results mean across three key areas impacting cardiovascular health: inflammation, hypertension, and hypercholesterolemia.

Pour Your Heart into It

If you want to prevent and reverse disease, slow the aging process, and be at your best, there is no more important place to put your attention and energy than your heart. It is both a symbol for love and compassion, and a finely engineered physical mechanism for living. Whichever way we choose to look at our heart, we must do our best to take care of it.

I've said that the root of all disease is inflammation, so let's start there.

Inflammation

A vast number of chronic health concerns, conditions, disorders, and diseases can be traced back to chronic cellular inflammation. Cellular inflammation occurs as a response to the presence of an unwanted substrate, such as a toxin, in the bloodstream. While it may be beneficial in short, acute instances to alert the body to dispatch the unwanted toxins, its continued occurrence over time leads to many chronic health conditions depending on the location of the inflammation in the body. The body has a built-in set of processes to manage and resolve inflammation. These processes are significantly influenced by the genes we carry in our DNA.

In the cardiovascular system, our chief area of concern is vascular inflammation, or inflammation that occurs in the blood vessels. Over time, chronic inflammation in the blood vessels can cause them to thicken and significantly reduce blood flow. This can increase your likelihood for an acute cardiovascular event such as a stroke or heart attack.

There are three conditions that influence your overall risk of cardiovascular inflammation, and they are as follows:

1. How well you remove toxins from your body before they can cause inflammation

This process involves the use of detoxification processes such as glutathionization and antioxidation. Glutathione is the major antioxidant of the body, and the efficiency with which it attaches to toxins and shuttles them to the liver for metabolism and removal is influenced by an important family of genes known as glutathione transferase. Three genes—GSTT1, GSTM1, and GSTP1—play a critical role in the coding of their respective enzymes, whose job is to attach glutathione to the toxin and render it harmless.

The GSTT1 and GSTM1 genes are tested as copy number variations because it is possible that you will be missing one or even both copies of these genes. In other words, you may not receive a copy from one or both of your parents, and as a result you don't have this gene at all in your DNA. This can significantly influence the efficiency of your body's detoxification capabilities. Ideally, you want to have both copies of both genes, and any reduction in the number of copies you have can reduce your overall detoxification capacity by as much as a combined 50 percent versus normal capacity.

The GSTP1 gene acts as a master glutathione gene and is involved in specifically removing toxins that cause health outcomes such as headaches, migraines, and brain fog. Examples of toxins targeted by the GSTP1 enzyme include polyaromatic hydrocarbons, cigarette smoke, heavy metals, chemicals, and pesticides.

Another important enzyme in your body is superoxide dismutase, whose job it is to remove harmful free radicals from the body before they can inflict cellular damage. The efficiency of your superoxide dismutase pathway depends on two genes: SOD2 and GPX. Together, these two genes produce enzymes that efficiently convert harmful oxidants into water and diatomic oxygen.

2. How well you respond at the cellular level when inflammation occurs

A cellular process known as methylation determines the efficiency with which your cells respond to the occurrence of inflammation. The more effective your overall methylation cycle, the better your cells will be at responding quickly and efficiently to mitigate the consequences of this inflammation. Methylation is also the process by which methyl groups are made available for the body to use. These methyl groups can be attached to toxins, which causes them to become harmless, more water-soluble, and thus easier to remove from the body. Several important genes, such as MTHFR, MTRR, MTR and SHMT1, play a role at different intervals of the cycle, but it is important to understand that it is the overall efficiency of the cycle and *not* the result of each individual gene that ultimately determines the efficiency of your anti-inflammatory and detoxification response.

3. The tolerance level of your blood vessels to the presence of toxins in the bloodstream

Your blood vessels provide blood to all the major organs in your body, including the heart and the brain. Naturally, it is important that inflammation in your blood vessels is quickly addressed, or else you risk potentially slowing down or completely stopping the flow of blood to these vital organs. The ability of your blood vessels to resist the impact of toxins in the bloodstream is significantly influenced by your DNA. An important chromosomal marker known as the 9P21 marker is strongly associated with optimal cardiovascular health. The number of G alleles you carry at this marker determines how resistant your blood vessels are to inflammation. The more Gs you carry, the less resistant you are and the more likely your blood vessels are to become inflamed. Chronically inflamed blood vessels thicken and can reduce or even completely stop the flow of blood to vital organs, which can increase your likelihood of an acute cardiovascular event such as a heart attack or a stroke.

The impact of your 9P21 can be mitigated if you carry specific versions of your 1P21 marker and PCSK9 gene. Specifically, carrying at least one G allele at your 1P21 marker and at least one T allele in your PCSK9 can significantly reduce your likelihood of cardiovascular disease.

Considering the questions I've asked about inflammation, here is a summary of my own possible health outcomes, based on my genetic tests:

I have an increased predisposition toward developing cardiovascular inflammation (a contributor to cardiovascular disease). Not a surprise, given my father's history, but a concern.

My body's defense against the onset of inflammation in my blood vessels caused by harmful toxins is suboptimal.

I have a suboptimal body environment profile. Several gene pathways influence your overall cardiovascular profile by determining how well you can remove toxins such as cigarette smoke, mold, oxidants, pollution, chemicals, and even estrogen metabolites from your body. This is important because too many toxins in your blood vessels can lead to inflammation, which can restrict blood flow and ultimately lead to health concerns like heart disease, high blood pressure, high cholesterol, stroke, and atherosclerosis (clogged arteries). Your cardiovascular system, like every system in your body, functions as a product of multiple processes, each with its own efficiencies. As a result, even if you have "good" versions of the cardiovascular genes like 9P21, APOE, and ACE, you could still be at a potentially increased risk for cardiovascular health concerns if processes like methylation, glutathionization, and antioxidation aren't working optimally.

Detoxification and Antioxidation

With my GSTT1 genotype, I have an average ability to remove toxins and harmful agents from my body.

I do not have the GSTM1 gene in my DNA. This means my ability to remove toxins and other harmful substances is significantly reduced.

Based on my GSTP1 genotype, I am more likely to manage and remove heavy metals from my body, as well as to resist sensory overload when it comes to strong smells and scents.

My SOD2 genotype enables me to quickly convert oxidants in the body into hydrogen peroxide via the superoxide dismutase pathway. While this is protective from an oxidant perspective, if I also carried a TT version of my GPX gene in combination with a CC version of my SOD2 gene, I would be more likely to see the graying and whitening of my hair occurring much earlier in life.

I convert hydrogen peroxide quickly into water and diatomic oxygen thanks to my GPX genotype. If you also have the TT version of the SOD2 gene, you may want to speak to your practitioner about monitoring your hydrogen peroxide levels to ensure you're maintaining appropriate levels.

Methylation

I am more likely to have optimal MTHFR and SHMT1 enzyme function.

I am also more likely to have suboptimal MTRR and MTR functioning. Because of my MTR genotype, I use adenosyl B_{12} instead of methyl B_{12} for my vitamin B_{12} supplementation.

I am more likely to have a suboptimal ability to absorb cofactors like vitamin B_{12}. That's why I take my B_{12} in a sublingual form that dissolves under the tongue.

Vascular

I have a normal risk of inflammation as well as cardiovascular health concerns.

I have a rare and beneficial version of the IP21 gene, which is associated with a reduced risk of cardiovascular disease and reduced levels of LDL cholesterol.

My PCSK9 genome is the most common and is associated with a normal risk of cardiovascular disease with no added protection.

Hypercholesterolemia

Hypercholesterolemia, also known as high cholesterol, is a chronic condition characterized by abnormally high levels of cholesterol in your blood. Cholesterol is a waxy substance used by the body for a number of important functions. In cardiovascular health, cholesterol's main function is to act as an anti-inflammatory agent at the site of inflammation. Important proteins known as lipoproteins shuttle cholesterol from the liver (where it is stored) to and from the site of inflammation. The proteins that transfer cholesterol *to* the site of inflammation are known as low-density lipoproteins (LDL). The proteins that transfer cholesterol *back* to the liver are known as high-density lipoproteins (HDL).

As a result of their function, high levels of LDL often are associated with suboptimal health outcomes because it means that the body is constantly shuttling cholesterol out to the sites of inflammation, but that cholesterol isn't coming back to the liver. This has given LDL a popular nickname as "bad" cholesterol and HDL as "good" cholesterol. However, the reality is that both proteins have specific functions to perform in the body.

What high levels of cholesterol *actually* indicate is that inflammation that is occurring in the body is not being effectively treated by cholesterol. One of the reasons this may occur is the increased presence of free radicals. Free radicals cause cholesterol to harden at the site of inflammation, which makes it more difficult for HDL to remove it and take it back to the liver. As a result, the liver keeps pumping out cholesterol at a faster rate than it is returned to the liver.

An important gene known as the APOE gene helps metabolize LDL efficiently. When this gene is not optimal, cholesterol buildup can occur much faster in your bloodstream, increasing your risk of high cholesterol. In general, the E2 (or "2") and E3 (or "3") versions of your APOE protein are healthier and more protective, while the E4 (or "4") version is more harmful. Since you receive one copy from each parent, the result you see below is a split between the version I received from my mother and the version I received from my father.

Your risk of high cholesterol can increase if you also carry a poor inflammatory, detoxification, and/or antioxidation response.

Here's how my APOE stacks up:

Gene/Gene Pathway	Result	Outcome
APOE	3/3	Optimal—Low Risk

Poor Response to Statins

Your SLCO1B1 gene controls statin metabolism. Statins are some of the most widely used medications on the planet. They reduce levels of LDL cholesterol in your body. The use of statins blocks cholesterol production but may also impact your ability to metabolize hormones such as testosterone, estrogen, vitamin D, and vitamin A. This may lead to nutritional deficiencies. If you experience muscle pain or fatigue from taking statins, talk to your doctor to determine if you need a blood test and your symptoms evaluated for statin-related nutritional deficiencies.

Like any other drug, the timing and dosing of your statins is based on generic clinical studies that determine how quickly/efficiently your body metabolizes and flushes out the statins you take. Your liver plays the primary role in this metabolism and ensures that you do not accumulate toxic/overdose levels of any medication (due to repeated daily doses). However, in a subset of the population, a suboptimal SLCO1B1 gene can mean that statins take much longer to be metabolized. This effectively imitates a drug overdose when taken day after day. An accumulated overdose of statihs can manifest as muscle pain and muscle fatigue (a condition known as *myopathy*). Left unaddressed, even more concerning liver toxicity and failure can occur.

My SLCO1B1 result:

Gene/Gene Pathway	Result	Outcome
SLCO1B1	T/T	Optimal—Low Risk

Hypertension

Hypertension, or high blood pressure, is defined as a chronic condition in which the blood vessels persistently experience periods of raised pressure. It is a dangerous condition when left unchecked, and it is often a major contributing factor in other, deadlier chronic diseases such as heart, brain, and kidney disease. Hypertension generally has a range from mild (early-morning headaches, nosebleeds, vision changes, and buzzing in the ears) to major symptoms (fatigue, nausea, chest pain, muscle tremors, and anxiety), but the arrival of any of these symptoms along with higher-than-normal readings for your blood pressure means the situation is already a serious one and shouldn't be taken lightly.

While every case of hypertension is different, in general hypertension is influenced by the following major factors: a diet high in salt and fats and low in fruits and vegetables, chronic stress, obesity, physical inactivity, consumption of alcohol and tobacco, family history, and genetics.

There are a number of functional genes that play an important role when it comes to your risk for hypertension.

Your ACE gene controls the version of angiotensin converting enzyme that your body produces. This enzyme is responsible for managing your body's blood pressure and salt reabsorption. It is sometimes known as the salt gene. If you have a more active version of this enzyme, you are more likely to have increased retention of salt and an increased constriction of your blood vessels. This increases the likelihood of having high blood pressure.

Note that your ethnicity can impact which allele of the ACE gene contributes to your risk of hypertension. If you have East Asian or South Asian ancestry, the A allele is considered the at-risk allele. If you come from European ancestry, the G allele is considered the at-risk allele. This is due to a phenomenon known as *epistasis*, which refers to the influence of two seemingly unrelated genes on each other based on your ethnicity.

Your NOS3 gene plays an important role in initiating dilation and constriction of your blood vessels. Just like it is important for your blood vessels to be "bulletproof," it is also important for them to be able to dilate and constrict on demand. When you exercise, your blood-flow requirements are increased. Ideally, your blood vessels should expand to compensate for the increased flow of blood. When your blood vessels are not able to dilate appropriately, there is a greater stress placed on important organs such as your heart and kidneys. This increased stress over years is one of the most important contributing factors to heart and kidney disease.

Your CLOCK gene manages your body's sleep-wake circadian rhythms. A proper sleep-wake cycle is essential to maintaining normal bodily processes that occur both during the day and while you sleep at night. Irregular sleep cycles that result in chronic poor sleep have been clinically linked to a higher risk of developing high blood pressure.

Your mood and behavioral genes can influence your risk of hypertension. While symptoms of anxiety aren't directly linked to long-term hypertension, they *can* cause temporary spikes in your blood pressure. When combined with the rest of your genetic and nongenetic factors, they can contribute to the overall symptoms of hypertension.

Your diet and nutrition genes can influence your relationships with fats, sugars, and insulin. A diet high in saturated fats and sugars can increase your risk of hypertension.

My results:

Gene/Pathway	Result	Meaning
ACE	A/A	Low risk of hypertension
CLOCK	T/T	Low risk of delayed and reduced sleep patterns
NOS3	G/G	Optimal nitric oxide response to vascular blood flow
Anxiety	Average Risk	Average risk for developing anxiety symptoms
Insulin Resistance	High Risk	High risk for developing insulin resistance based on diet choices

Optimal cardiovascular health is a critical aspect of optimal human health and longevity. Cardiovascular disease is the number one cause of death in the world. However, it is a chronic disease, which means it doesn't occur suddenly but instead develops over time.

By understanding your genetic profile and being proactive about reducing your risk of inflammation—a major root cause of all chronic disease—you can take significant steps in not only preserving but optimizing your cardiovascular health throughout your life.

I encourage you to take a multidisciplinary approach to ensure optimal cardiovascular health by personalizing your diet, nutrition, lifestyle, environment, and supplementation according to your unique genomic profile.

In other words—*pour your heart into it!*

To get better insights into my cardiovascular health, my team suggested that I get regular blood tests done to track changes in the following:

- Cholesterol profile (includes total cholesterol, LDL, HDL, and triglycerides)
- Homocysteine
- Hemoglobin A1c
- Vitamin D
- C-reactive protein
- erythrocyte sedimentation rate

Since the only element of my cardiovascular profile that could potentially pose a problem for me is inflammation, I'll share some of the suggestions I received. If I had had an issue with hypertension, high cholesterol, or other problems, I would share them here. I'm purposely not sharing what the suggestions *might* be because I once again want to make the point that the suggestions you receive are only as good as the insights you get from your unique test results.

Here are some of the things I'm doing to combat my propensity for inflammation.

Lifestyle

- Meet with a nutritionist or health coach to design meals that meet the diet and nutrition needs outlined above.
- Source and purchase an organic and/or biodynamic olive oil to add to your food daily (1 to 2 tablespoons daily).
- Buy a pedometer so you can track your daily steps.
- Set up your bedroom so you sleep in a completely dark and cool environment.

Habits to Adopt

- Remove packaged, processed, and high-sodium foods from your diet.
- Incorporate foods high in antioxidants—berries, cacao, matcha green tea, and pecans, for example.
- Completely remove alcohol, sugars, and fried foods from your diet.
- Portion at least 50 percent of your plate with high-fiber green vegetables (at least 25 g). For example, you could eat organic spinach with your lunch each day.
- Drink green tea twice a day between meals.
- Practice deep-breathing exercises before each meal (aim for 5 minutes of breathing about three times a day).

Behaviors to Avoid

- Eating foods that contain preservatives and food coloring. In addition, don't eat processed foods and fast food.
- Eating fried foods.
- Smoking (including e-cigarettes and hookah/shisha).
- Excessive consumption of simple carbohydrates, such as bread, pasta, and rice.
- Excessive consumption of alcohol.

Supplements

- Mitochondrial Optimizer
- Methylation Optimizer
- Detox Optimizer
- Vitamin D
- Omega-3
- Coenzyme-Q10

Chapter 8

DNA, HORMONES, FITNESS, AND BODY TYPE

Hormones get no respect. We think of them as the elusive chemicals that make us a bit moody, but these magical little molecules do so much more.

— SUSANNAH CAHALAN, JOURNALIST AND AUTHOR OF *BRAIN ON FIRE*

If you were a fan of comic books when you were a kid, as I was, you may remember the ads for products and services that were being hawked inside. They were the staples of a boy's life—X-ray specs to help you see through clothing and walls, kits for model airplanes and boats, toy soldier collections, air rifles and BB guns, video games, sea monkeys, and more.

Since I couldn't afford the comic books or any of the products being advertised inside them, I read them on the rack at the grocery store until someone shooed me away. Or I read them in the homes of my friends. Or I read them if the books had been thrown away. It didn't matter where they were, I craved those stories. And although there was an endless supply of heroes and villains, the one constant was those advertisements.

After reading stories about having superheroes with powers of every sort, kids were easy targets for products and services that promised to bring them closer to having their own superpowers—at least earthly ones. One popular ad genre was for building muscles. Which makes sense because how else were you going to become Thor or Captain America or Batman?

There was one from a guy named "Mike Marvel" who wore Tarzan-like trunks and had women fawning over him as he pitched his "patented and secret Dynaflex method" that claimed he could build you a "magnificent new He-Man-muscled body in just ten minutes a day—with absolutely NO weights—NO bar-bells—NO EXERCISE AT ALL!" for $1.98.

Another ad featured a smiling young gap-toothed and absurdly proportioned future actor and governor named Arnold Schwarzenegger selling the Joe Weider system. In the ad, the seven-time Mr. Olympia bodybuilding champion said he "put 2 full inches on my arms, 3 inches on my chest and trimmed 4 inches off my waist in just 7 weeks," and asked, "Why not you?" In his photo he's wearing only tiny shorts, with his left arm he's lifting a beautiful bikini-clad woman up in the air as she holds aloft the Weider system's pamphlets, and he's flexing his 22-inch biceps on his right arm. This system was said to be "FREE," with some fine print underneath.

But the longest-running and most successful advertising campaign of this kind was for the Dynamic Tension program offered by Charles Atlas (born Angelo Siciliano in Acri, Italy, in 1892). The comic-strip ad—headlined "The Insult That Made a Man Out of Mac"—depicted a beach scene featuring a bully kicking sand in the face of a "weakling" named Mac who was with his girl. This caused the skinny guy to vow to gain a more "manly" physique so he could take on the bully. Weeks after ordering the Atlas Dynamic Tension program, the formerly weak and now muscled-up Mac goes back to the bully on the beach and punches him in the mouth with his girl looking on admiringly. While I believe the Atlas company stopped running the ads in printed comic books many years ago, they still do business online, raking in more than half a million dollars in annual revenue.

And it wasn't just ads targeting boys. They preyed on female insecurities as well. There were ads for losing weight, getting the boy or man of your dreams, and even increasing bust size. One such ad for the Mark Eden Developer claimed that by using the product for one week, customers could increase their bust size by three inches.

The product consisted of two connected pieces of plastic shaped like clam shells with a spring inside, and an instruction booklet. The copy inside is, well, revealing. "So many women who have been literally 'flat as boards' have achieved higher, fuller, lovelier bust-lines in a remarkably short time with the Mark Eden method. And a woman whose bustline is suddenly transformed from the average or below average to a richer fuller development receives more for her efforts than just a larger reading on the tape measure. She is subtly transformed as a woman. There is an incomparable difference in the entire feminine line, shape, and grace of her whole figure. Her very presence takes on a new and subtle glow of womanliness, of sex-appeal, and yes, of glamour that is undeniable and unmistakable."

You will be shocked to know that the Mark Eden Bust Developer did not quite live up to its claims. After being accused of 11 counts of mail fraud, it was taken off the market. However, not before selling 18,000 of the gadgets at $9.95 each.

I tell you this not only because it's impossible for any of these snake-oil solutions to work as advertised, but also because they take unhealthy shortcuts and ignore the interdependence of hormones, body type, and fitness in achieving outcomes. Unless you understand your DNA and what it's telling you, you will waste a lot of time and money and effort on get-fit-quick solutions being peddled by unscrupulous hucksters.

And you will never know the actual superpowers that exist within you.

Let's look at how body type, hormones, and fitness go together.

Body Type

We have different perspectives on what we want from body types and what our goals are. That's fair for everybody. What you want is what you should aim for. But how do you get there unless you understand genetically what your body's designed to be?

This is hormonally driven. The estrogen and testosterone in your body, which are genetically predetermined, will define what you look like outwardly. And if you're striving and working hard toward a specific goal but you don't know what you're wired to be, you may be wasting your time or even hurting yourself. This is where it becomes important to decode the hormones of your genetics and understand what your dominant hormone is. Whether you're a man or a woman.

There's a woman for whom it doesn't matter what you do, you can't get the shape, you can't get the curves. You're testosterone or androgen dominant. You can get the six-pack abs without even trying, but you can't get the hips.

There's a woman for whom the hips and the curves are no problem. But try and get those defined and striated muscles, and it never happens. This is hormonally based, and it's true for men and women.

There's a man for whom it doesn't matter how hard you train, you can get big, you can get strong, but you can't get ripped. There are men who can get strong, and they can get ripped, but they can't get big.

These are challenges we're facing as we reach for our goals, and we're using one-size-fits-all-type applications to get there when that's not how the human body works.

When you understand your genetics, you at least understand, foundationally, what your body is wired to do—what hormones are telling your systems and how you are designed, physically. From there, it's much easier to set your goals and decide what to do next.

Weight Management

The one area where the failure of one-size-fits-all applications has touched almost all of us is in weight management. This is where we ask, What do I eat? How do I train? How do I burn fat? How do I add muscle?

The one-size-fits-all answers don't work for most of us because most of us aren't wired the same way. We need unique solutions.

It starts with the brain, and how we perceive food, satiety, bingeing, addiction, leaning on food as a coping mechanism. That's already hardwired into our brains.

You then get to personalized diet and nutrition. How do I deal with fats? How do I deal with carbs? How do I deal with macro- and micronutrients in general?

The important foundation to it all is based on your hormones. If you don't understand how you're hormonally designed, you can't understand how you deal with fat. For the women who are constantly trying to deal with cellulite, dealing with the symptoms as opposed to understanding hormonally why it's even happening, imagine the implications of constantly fighting only the first layer of that battle. How frustrating and demoralizing that must be.

This is true for weight management in general. When it comes to storing fat, not having enough muscle, knowing how to add more muscle—it is all hormonally driven. And understanding your hormones will tell you how you are wired to do these things. But more important, for the changes you are seeking, how do you do it for yourself? Not the one-size-fits-all, not the trial and error, but what works for you.

Hair Loss

One thing that comes up a lot in our business is the genetics of hair loss, how there must be some correlation. And of course, there is. It's not the stories you hear about how hair loss comes from the mom's side or the dad's side or how it skips a generation. Yes, it's a genetic inheritance. It's a legacy of your parents and it's passed on to you. But it's rooted in one thing: dihydrotestosterone (DHT). It's a potent, manly man version of testosterone that is also responsible for giving you those ripped, striated muscles.

The toxicity of DHT is what leads to that follicle death and eventual hair loss. The beauty is that by testing a five-year-old child, you can know decades in advance if their hormonal pathway will lead to hair loss, whether they're a boy or a girl.

In health care, there's another issue that sticks out as highly important: prostate enlargement. The same toxic DHT, that manly man testosterone that leads to follicle death, also leads to prostate enlargement, which of course we all want to avoid. But the good news is by knowing this early, you can do something about it.

So again, for men and women, understanding hair loss comes down to understanding hormones. Am I rich in DHT? If I am, I'm no longer rich in hair. Or am I rich in estrogen, with that thick, full, beautifully flowing hair, whether I'm a man or a woman? Understanding your hormone profile will enable you to know what you need to do about hair loss and hair retention.

Female Hormones

With patients we've dealt with in person in our clinic, the area where we see the biggest room for improvement in the delivery of health care is female hormone health.

Stuff that is black-and-white at the genetic level has been treated as gray. It's unfortunate that it's been taken for granted that these problems are just meant to happen: it's "your hormones," and you have no choice but to suffer through it. Things like menopause, fibromyalgia, fertility issues—they're not understood at the root-cause level and therefore they're only treated at the symptom level.

We've come to understand many things in this area. First, hormones are not the same for all women. Estrogen metabolism, testosterone metabolism, estrogen toxicity—these are factors that are not considered. Are you estrogen dominant, meaning you are genetically wired to behave and physically manifest as more feminine? Are you androgen or testosterone dominant, where it's hard for you to get that curvaceous figure, and you have those firm, ripped muscles, but fertility, polycystic ovary syndrome (PCOS), and other issues may arise because of the imbalance in your hormones?

This is where we've gone deep genetically and mapped out the hormonal cascade so we understand what that looks like for you. Breast health, menopause, fertility, even puberty—all these things that women go through that are treated as gray can be made black-and-white if you look at them through a personalized genetic lens.

Male Hormones

Men are more likely than women to ignore their health and leave it for a later date, playing superhero and trying to get through. And one area where we see this is in hormone health, which gets completely ignored.

There are areas like libido, hair loss, and prostate health where you don't start to deal with them until it's too late. This is where, by understanding your hormone health early on, you can begin to map out your future and understand what to do well ahead of time.

If you're concerned about prostate health, if you're concerned about longevity and maintaining that high level of testosterone, which is the single greatest marker for longevity, you first must understand how you deal with hormones. What if you're estrogen dominant? What if that hormone replacement therapy the doctor gives you to boost your levels gets converted into estrogen because that's what you do at a genetic level? You need to understand this before you can start to get into solutions.

That is why we believe that all men, just like women, need to pay attention to their hormones to understand the major male issues— the things you want to know about, like hair loss and libido, and the things you don't want to know about, like prostate health and longevity. Decode the map, understand your hormones, and ensure you have vitality for life.

Hormones and Fitness

To truly understand fitness, you must know your hormones. To get away from trial-and-error, one-size-fits-all solutions, you need to know what works for you. And that's done by understanding how your body is wired. How is it designed? What was it meant to look like? It's only then that you can understand what you're designed to do. Without that understanding you end up putting a load on your system that causes the wrong things to happen, that leads to health care implications. As you go through the genetics of your hormone system, you'll start to discover how you're wired, how you're mapped, and what proper decisions to make.

In the next section I'll cover the genes that influence the production and balance of your hormones. As usual, I'll reveal my own test results and what they mean for me.

Your Real Superpower

My favorite superhero was Batman.

By the time he was 18 years old he had mastered nutrition, biomechanics, training, and weightlifting. He used technology that made Tony Stark look like a Luddite. He had a genius-level IQ, could speak 15 languages, and had advanced degrees in biology, math, technology, physics, mythology, geography, history, criminal science, forensic science, computer science, engineering, and chemistry. He could run as fast as Usain Bolt; he had mastered 127 different forms of martial arts; he could bench-press 1,000 pounds, military press 600 pounds, and curl 350 pounds; he had a lung capacity so great he could hold his breath underwater for seven minutes, and with his bare hands he once caught an arrow shot at his head.

Unlike his arch nemesis, Deathstroke, who was an artificially enhanced meta-human due to an advanced hormone treatment program, Batman was all natural. He wanted to prevent and reverse crime, make it possible for people to live longer, and help the citizens of Gotham optimize their performance in all aspects of life. He had to face some dark internal demons in his psyche—fear, self-destructiveness, and self-pity among them—but he did it and became a superhero in the process.

Batman couldn't fly without a plane, burn holes through steel without a laser beam, or stop a locomotive without using its brakes, but he was the best superhero to me because he was more realistic in what he could do. Genetically, he was just like you or me—a normal human. But I saw the larger message of what he was about—improve yourself, improve the world—and it gave me something to strive for in my own way.

If Batman had one superpower, it was his drive to acquire knowledge and put it to good use.

So, in the spirit of Batman, let's do some of that.

There are three major classes of hormones: progesterone, androgens like testosterone, and estrogens. The unique combination of genetic variations in your genes will influence your hormone levels and impact things like your body type and your ability to lose weight and put on muscle, as well as gender-based health concerns.

In males, hormone imbalance can influence your risk of health concerns like balding, cystic acne, weight gain, gynecomastia (developing larger male breasts), prostate enlargement, low libido, and poor sexual function.

In females, hormone imbalance can influence your risk of health concerns such as PCOS, endometriosis, fibroids, infertility, menopause symptoms, premenstrual syndrome symptoms, and even breast and ovarian cancers.

Similar to the methylation cycle, it is important that you evaluate your hormone profile based on the entire hormone pathway and not just the results for each individual gene. Otherwise, you may find that individual gene results don't quite match up with your outward physical appearance or health concerns.

Hormone production and management has two steps. The first step is steroidogenesis, which is how hormones are produced. The second step is more relevant to females than males and deals with estrogen metabolism.

The following breakdown of genes is designed to give you an understanding of the function of each gene, and how the roles those genes play influences the overall result when it comes to your hormone profile.

Androgens and estrogens are the two major categories of sex hormones produced by humans. Many areas of your health and wellness are influenced by these sex hormones, including growth, sexual maturity, reproduction, and overall longevity.

Your genes influence the production of your sex hormones, which contributes to your overall health and well-being.

Here are my own test results:

Gene Tested	CYP17A1	SRD5A2	ANDROx	CYP19A1	UGT2B17	UGT2B15	GSTP1	GPX
Result	GG	CG	CC	CC	1	TT	AA	CC

Gene Tested	CYP1A1	CYP1B1	CYP3A4	NOS3	9P21	SOD2	GSTT1 (copies)	GSTM1 (copies)
Result	AA	CC	AA	GG	3G	CC	1	0

These results indicate that I am androgen dominant. This means I tend to produce high levels of hormones in general, but particularly higher levels of androgens like testosterone and DHT than estrogens. Androgen-dominant males like me are more likely to have an easier time putting on and keeping lean, defined muscle mass (the "cut" look); to have an overall leaner frame; to have an increased resistance to weight and fat gain; to be less likely to develop cellulite; to have a greater potential for increased insulin resistance; to have a larger prostate; to have a more defined jawline and prominent Adam's apple; to develop cystic acne, thinning hair, and male pattern balding; and to have an excess of body or facial hair. If you've seen a photo or video of me, you'll notice those characteristics fit me perfectly.

Androgen-dominant females are more likely to have irregular periods, an increased risk of PCOS, and smaller breasts and narrower hips.

Genes That Influence My Genotype

My genotype is associated with fast CYP17A1 function. As a result, I convert progesterone into testosterone at a faster rate. This means I generally produce increased levels of sex hormones and am more likely to carry a dominant hormone profile.

I carry the genotype associated with increased androgen binding to the androgen receptor. This means my androgens (like testosterone and DHT) bind more efficiently to their receptors. As a result,

154

I'm more likely to see characteristics associated with higher levels of androgens. For instance, I am more likely to quickly put on lean muscle mass as well as to keep it on for longer.

I have a slow version of CYP19A1. This means I convert testosterone into estrogen at a slower rate and I am more likely to have lower levels of estrogen.

The SRD5A2 gene controls the rate at which the body converts testosterone into DHT. DHT is five times more potent in its androgenizing properties than testosterone. As I said earlier, high levels of DHT are strongly associated with male pattern balding, hair thinning, and excess body hair. I convert testosterone into DHT at a medium rate, and I am more likely to have normal levels of DHT.

I have one copy of the UGT2B17 gene, which indicates normal gene functioning. Along with the UGT2B15 and CYP3A4 genes, UGT2B17 is responsible for metabolizing and clearing out androgens like testosterone and DHT via a process known as *glucuronidation*, which removes hormones via urine and bile.

My genotype is associated with fast UGT2B15 functioning. This means I clear out androgens like testosterone and DHT at a faster rate than other people, which may lead to reduced androgen levels in my body.

Genes That Influence Fitness, Rest, and Recovery

The genotype I have has a normal amount of resistance to vascular inflammation. This means my body is more likely to respond normally to increased levels of oxidants produced during high-intensity or long-duration periods of cardiovascular exercise. However, pushing my body over time at higher intensities or durations may lead to inflammation in my endothelial lining if I don't provide it with enough rest and antioxidants through my diet and nutrition choices. As in every case of my test results, whether I'm normal, below normal, or above normal is one thing; the load I put on it is another thing.

My genotype indicates that I have an optimal nitric oxide response to vascular blood flow. I can engage in moderate amounts of cardiovascular exercise along with weightlifting exercises. I am more likely to have normal vasodilation (relaxing of my blood vessels) as a result of normal nitric oxide levels.

My body does not respond well to toxins such as oxidants, chemicals from the environment, or infections. This was proven to be true when we were first building our offices and my body could not adequately process all the toxic insults it was receiving. In addition, I take longer to recover from periods of exercise, particularly strenuous or lengthy workout sessions. I am also more likely to experience extended periods of fatigue, muscle soreness, tiredness, and lack of energy as a result.

According to my test results, my body can address high levels of oxidants in an efficient manner and also is more likely to have optimal mitochondrial function. This means that if I do the right things, I should recover at a normal pace following periods of exercise.

Superhero Health and Beauty Regimen

Many forms of exercise are beneficial for humans, but the length, intensity, and choice of exercise you engage in should vary depending on your unique genomic profile. In addition, the diet you choose and the length of time you need to recover from a workout also play important roles. In this section, I will address some important questions to ask when beginning an optimized fitness and exercise regimen, as well as break down the recommendations I received in this regard.

What Kind of Workout Is Best for *Me*?

Your sex hormones play an important role in shaping your overall optimal fitness profile. Androgens like testosterone and DHT promote fat metabolism and muscle growth, while estrogens promote fat storage. In both males and females, the unique balance of sex hormones can influence how easy or difficult it can be to physically resemble an optimal fitness profile. Note, however, that one does not have to *look* healthy to *be* healthy. On top of this, your body's response to the oxidants produced during intense or lengthy exercise sessions should also influence which type of exercise you engage in the most to reduce the risk of injury caused by excessive exercise.

Rest and Recovery

Rest and recovery are often overlooked or misunderstood but are incredibly important aspects of an optimal fitness and workout protocol. Like any well-oiled machine, the body requires a period of downtime to rest and recover from extended periods of intense use.

During workouts, your body burns through energy and oxygen at a much faster and more intense rate than normal. As a result, you build up by-products like lactic acid and oxidants at much faster rates as well. When you rest and recover, you allow your body to execute important recovery processes like antioxidation, detoxification, energy replenishment, muscle and tissue repair, and cellular repair. Your unique genomic profile significantly influences your ability to perform these important processes.

My Workout

Based on my genomic profile, here are some recommendations I received and reviewed with my health care provider and physical trainer. I can't say this enough: *never* begin a workout regimen without prior discussion with your health care provider. I also strongly recommend hiring a physical trainer to help you learn the best way to perform effective exercises to reach your goals.

My mix of strength training and cardiovascular training should be 70 percent to 30 percent, respectively.

Strength training: Avoid doing multiple reps at my maximum weight for any exercise. Follow a general rule of heavier weights, but fewer repetitions per exercise.

Cardiovascular: Exercise at no more than 60 percent of my maximum heart rate. I should be able, with a little difficulty, to have a conversation with someone while working out.

Workout Breakdown

Strength training: Up to three days per week. No more than 45 minutes per workout. Rotate between exercises for different muscle groups every day.

Cardiovascular: No more than two days per week. No more than 45 minutes per workout.

Rest and Recovery

Ensure seven to eight hours of sleep a day and at least two days of rest between workouts. Use the sauna frequently to support reduced recovery times.

When Is the Best Time to Work Out?

The function of your sex hormones is based on circadian rhythms. Estrogens function on a monthly cycle (commonly known as the menstrual cycle), while androgens function on a daily cycle. While the best time to work out depends on your goals, the following rules can be generally applied for the most optimal performance for each sex.

Males

Males have a significant daily circadian rhythm when it comes to their sex hormones, particularly testosterone. Testosterone shares a direct inverse relationship with cortisol—the testosterone level rises when the cortisol level drops, and vice versa. As males age, their overall testosterone level decreases, so it's important to take advantage of the times when it is at its highest to get the best return on investment in workouts.

Strength Training

Testosterone peaks between the hours of 6 and 8 A.M. as well as 4 and 6 P.M. Ideally, this is when you will experience the most explosive performance when it comes to strength and weight training. If you feel significantly hungry after workouts, stick to working out in the evening to reduce the risk of overeating throughout the day.

Cardio

Best in the evenings, shortly after 6 P.M. Running in the evening reduces the risk of injury to muscles that are otherwise stiff in the morning. It also prevents you from overeating all day and can be a great way to reduce stress. Finally, it can improve your ability to fall asleep if you struggle with poor sleep.

Females

Estrogens play a far more important role in the female body than the male body. As a result, menstruating females should pay closer attention to the time of the month when it comes to the type and intensity of exercise in which they engage.

Assuming Day 1 is the first day of your period, consider the following breakdown when it comes to planning your exercises.

Days 1 to 10 (the Follicular Phase)

Studies show this is the best time to engage in strength training and weightlifting.

Schedule your heaviest, toughest, and highest-endurance exercises during this period.

Days 11 to 16 (Ovulation)

As the estrogen level rises, the risk of injury, particularly to tendons, increases. During this period, ensure that you allocate extra time for warm-up, stretching, and cool-down exercises during your workouts.

Days 17 to 28 (the Luteal Phase)

During the second part of your cycle, your progesterone level rises to its highest, with a simultaneous drop in estrogen level.

This can significantly impact your endurance and performance, so don't be surprised if you're not performing at your usual level during this phase.

In this period, focus on maintenance over gains. Avoid pushing yourself to the max. This is a great time to take extra rest and recovery days and prepare yourself for your next strength-training cycle.

Menopausal and Postmenopausal Females

Recommendations for menopausal and postmenopausal women will differ based on several factors, including their hormone dominance, workout goals, and lifestyle and nutrition choices. Discuss the right workout plan with a personal trainer who can understand your personal situation before placing you on a protocol.

For general muscle-building and maintenance, consider weight-lifting and resistance-based exercises.

Monitor your heart rate during periods of cardiovascular exercise to ensure you aren't pushing yourself too hard.

Avoid doing intense exercises too early in the morning or too late in the evening, as both are associated with an increased risk of muscle injury.

Hair Health

Hair serves a number of important roles depending on where it is found on the body. Your relationships with hair growth, development, and maturity are strongly related to the balance of your sex hormones, which are strongly associated with your genomic profile.

In this section, I'll look at hair-related health outcomes that are influenced by your sex hormone profile.

Hair Thinning, Hair Loss, and Male Pattern Balding

As I said earlier, based on my genotype, I am more likely to experience symptoms associated with hair thinning, hair loss, or male pattern balding. All I needed was a mirror to tell me that, but my genetic test told me *why* and highlighted some other issues that could arise.

Hair thinning and balding is a health outcome that can be attributed to a combination of many factors. Hormone balance plays an important role in your predisposition for hair loss. As a result, your genetics can predict to some degree how likely you are to experience hair-related concerns.

In general, an individual with a higher ratio of androgens to estrogens is more likely to experience hair thinning and loss, a receding hairline, and/or balding. Research has shown that a combination of increased androgen receptors on your hair follicles, a higher level of DHT production, and a higher level of testosterone all predispose your hair follicles to a shorter growth phase (known as the anagen) and a longer resting phase (known as the telogen). The longer your follicles remain in telogen, the less anchored your hair is to your scalp and the easier it is for your hair to fall out.

Hirsutism

I am more likely to see the development and persistence of excessive body and facial hair growth. Again, the mirror does not lie!

Surprisingly, the same high levels of androgens that can increase your risk of losing the hair on your scalp can *increase* the hair production on other parts of your body. *Hirsutism* is defined as the excessive growth of body and facial hair. This is usually depicted as thick, coarse, and dark hair that grows in places where lighter and thinner hair would normally grow—such as above the lips and on the back or lower abdomen, as well as the arms and legs. While the exact reason for this is unclear, what is known is that higher levels of androgens play an important role in increasing your likelihood of excessive body and facial hair growth.

Skin Health

The skin is the largest organ of the human body. Skin health is often associated with cosmetics. However, like any organ, skin requires an optimal relationship between diet, lifestyle, environment, and genetics to remain healthy.

Sex hormones play an important role in your overall skin health. The balance of your hormones influences the production of skin oils, the depositing of fat underneath your skin (known as *cellulite*), and the strength, flexibility, healing, and barrier functioning of your skin.

In this section, I'll explore common skin health concerns associated with sex hormones.

Cystic Acne

Based on my genotype, I am more likely to experience symptoms associated with cystic acne. I am far from alone, as we see many people in our clinic with this issue.

Cystic acne is a severe form of acne in which cysts form beneath the skin due to a combination of bacteria, oil, and dry skin cells that get trapped in your pores. Acne is a common occurrence in teens as they begin to produce sex hormones. Severe cases of acne, like cystic acne, continue into adulthood and are much more painful and inflammatory than common acne.

A major contributor to occurrences of cystic acne is hormonal imbalance. Specifically, individuals with higher levels of androgens, such as those classified as androgen- or co-dominant, seem to have a greater predisposition toward cystic acne. Higher levels of testosterone increase the body's production of sebum, which is the oil that prevents the skin from drying out.

Cellulite

My genes indicate that I am less likely to develop cellulite. Cellulite is a relatively harmless skin condition that occurs because of the accumulation of fat cells between the fibrous cords that hold your skin together. This results in the appearance of dimpling and uneven surfaces across the skin, particularly around areas of larger fat deposits. Cellulite occurs at a much higher rate in women than in men due to its association with estrogen. It is significantly influenced by the balance of your sex hormones, which is why it generally tends to show up after puberty. As a result, your unique genomic profile plays an important role in your predisposition to develop cellulite. While weight gain can make cellulite more noticeable, cellulite also can occur in lean individuals.

The sex hormone estrogen plays an important role in your predisposition for cellulite. Because of its association with fat storage, an imbalance in estrogen levels can lead to excessive fat storage as a response. Individuals who are estrogen dominant tend to be most likely to see cellulite development. As I've said, I am androgen dominant.

Lifestyle

- Hire a personal trainer to design a strength-training workout for you and learn proper form.
- Go through your workout clothes and purge the ones that don't fit.
- Fill your social feed with inspiring influencers who focus on the science of fitness, not just looks and aesthetics.
- Learn about heart-rate thresholds and what it feels like at different rates.
- Find a workout buddy to join you on a strength-training regimen.
- Join a local running or walking club.
- Purchase an air purifier for your home or office.
- Install blackout curtains and a white-noise machine in your bedroom.
- Set up a corner of your home with a yoga mat, block, and relaxation pillow.
- Get rid of common household cleaners, air fresheners, and toiletries and replace them with organic options.

Habits to Adopt

- Put on your gym clothes at the same time every day, even if you don't intend to exercise.
- Get a committed workout buddy for your weightlifting workouts.
- After you start the kettle for tea, do squats until the water boils. Get your body used to moving.
- Watch fitness-related shows and videos on Netflix.
- Dance after dinner each night while you clean up (kids love this!).
- Hang out with people who are already exercising in the ways you admire.
- Eat antioxidant-rich foods at every meal: berries, citrus fruits, and leafy greens, for example.
- Turn on the air purifier in your bedroom in the evening, just before getting in bed.
- Take hot baths or sauna visits multiple times each week.
- Buy natural cleaning products that are free from perfumes and polychlorinated aromatic hydrocarbons (PCAHs).

Behaviors to Avoid

- Using time-wasting apps such as social media or games on your phone.
- Hitting the Snooze button—get up and get to that workout!
- Grazing for snacks all evening.
- Making other appointments a priority over your fitness—this is your long-term health we're talking about.
- Watching TV while sitting instead of while actively moving.

Supplements for building muscle

- L-carnitine
- Whey or vegan protein isolate

Supplements for rest and recovery

- N-acetylcysteine (NAC)
- Selenium
- Milk thistle
- BCAA (branched-chain amino acids)
- Tocotrienols
- Coenzyme Q10

Hair Health

Lifestyle

- Purchase high-quality fenugreek teas and spices.
- Clear your home of toxic cleaning products and toiletries.
- Ask your clinician if a tocotrienol supplement is a good idea for you.
- Collect recipes that use fenugreek in them.

Habits to Adopt

- Purchase cleaning products and toiletries that are packaged in glass bottles.
- Only use hair products with naturally derived ingredients.
- Wear clothing and accessories that highlight the aspects of your hair and body that you like best.
- Consider a DHT blocker to slow hair loss.

Always speak to a specialist clinician before trying any hairgrowth products. Usually, it takes a combination of many different solutions to help your hair grow back—your clinician will be able to provide you with the best guidance.

Behaviors to Avoid

- Using household products with harsh chemicals that can disrupt your hormone balance.

- Using excessive testosterone (TRT) and other forms of hormone replacement therapy for muscle growth without understanding your genetic risks.
- Using hair growth or elimination products that aren't evidence-based.

Supplements

- Saw palmetto
- Lycopene
- Fenugreek
- Zinc
- Green tea extract (EGCG)
- Diindolylmethane (DIM)
- Indole-3-carbinol (I3C)
- Resveratrol
- Male A hormone support

Skin Health—Cystic Acne

Lifestyle

- Schedule a check-up with your dermatologist and present your genetic report showing them your propensity for higher DHT levels.
- Get rid of plastic bottles and containers and household cleaners with heavy chemicals.
- Purchase a round of natural essential oils packaged in glass bottles.
- Talk to your dermatologist about reducing your usage of any skincare products that have strong drying agents (that reduce sebum production). This might include anything with retinoids, antiandrogens, or antibiotics.
- Replace your laundry detergent with a hypoallergenic, sensitive-skin, fragrance-free detergent.

Habits to Adopt

- Drink a cup of fenugreek tea each day.
- Follow a structured skincare routine (morning and evening).
- Read the labels before you purchase new home/body products.
- Add healthy fats to your diet: avocados, coconuts, olive oil.
- Cleanse your skin immediately after excessive sweating or using natural sunscreen.

Behaviors to Avoid

- Buying products packaged in plastic bottles.
- Consuming dairy products (milk, yogurt, cheese, etc.)—at least for a few weeks. Alternatives are widely available.
- Picking at the acne on your face (it's tempting, but oh so harmful).

Supplements

- Saw palmetto
- Lycopene
- Fenugreek
- Zinc
- Green tea extract (EGCG)
- Diindolylmethane (DIM)
- Indole-3-carbinol (I3C)
- Resveratrol
- Male A hormone support
- Female A hormone support

Chapter 9

DNA, INFLAMMATION, IMMUNITY, AND DETOX

By cleansing your body on a regular basis and eliminating as many toxins as possible from your environment, your body can begin to heal itself, prevent disease, and become stronger and more resilient than you ever dreamed possible!

— DR. EDWARD GROUP III, FOUNDER AND CEO AT GLOBAL HEALING

In everything I do—food, travel, movement, anything—I plan around how those things are going to affect my health. For instance, if I know I'm going to be having dinner with a business partner, I will try to have a say in where we'll eat. If I can't do that, I'll check out the menu online before I even get there so I can be more comfortable making an informed and healthy choice. If I'm going to an unfamiliar city, I will check the air quality and try to stay in a hotel that has a record of being clean and healthy. If I'm exercising or simply getting up from a chair, I pay attention to my biomechanics so I don't injure myself in any way.

To some, this may sound obsessive, like I'm afraid to live. But to me, it's being mindful about my health, like it's a hobby in which I am heavily invested. I'm competing with myself to see just how healthy I can be. Why do I do this?

Each day, my body, like yours, is exposed to a variety of external and internal stressors, such as viral or bacterial infections, internal toxins such as estrogen metabolites or free radicals, chemicals, and other environmental agents. These stressors cause inflammation, which is the root cause of all illness. It's hard enough for my body to address the myriad causes and outcomes related to inflammation, so the least I can do is to protect my anti-inflammatory, immune, and detoxification systems so they can fight off these stressors.

Protection starts with evaluation, with knowing what kind of anti-inflammatory abilities I have, and proper evaluation begins with getting my genome tested. It does for you too. But before I get to the genetic pathways involved in our anti-inflammation, immunity, and detoxification systems—and share my own genetic test results in this area—I want to talk about how we approach this topic in our research and with our clinical practitioners.

Immunity and Detox

We pair immunity with detox because we know there's a functional layer that the conversation about health has been missing. When we think about immunity, we know that there are white blood cells out there fighting off viruses and bacteria, trying to keep us healthy. Think of those white blood cells as our soldiers fighting to protect us.

Where detox is implicit in this is the battleground. When you have cells that are already under stress from external and internal forces and you add on top of that a layer of virus or a bacterial insult, the outcome is different for each person. If one person is healthy at the cellular level and another person is unhealthy at the cellular level, how and to what degree they get sick will be different. This is what we look at as we explore immunity and detox.

Detoxification

So, what is detoxification? We hear this word thrown around a lot, but what does it mean and how does it work? There's a process called *glutathionization* where glutathione is deployed in the body to bind to toxins and take them to the liver, where the toxins are then metabolized and cleared from your system.

At a genetic level, it's possible to not even have the genetic instruction for this process because you never got a copy of the GSTT1 and the GSTM1 genes from your mom and dad in your genetic code. That means your body can't properly execute the process of glutathionization. You could be doing it at 20 to 30 percent capacity versus someone who is at full capacity. It's not that you're doing anything wrong; it's simply the genetic hand you were dealt.

Now, if you're exposed to the things that are putting toxins into your body—environmentally, nutritionally, or because of a lifestyle choice—what would the net result be? The answer is inflammation.

Inflammation

When you put a load on your cells and they're under stress from toxic insults, damage is done. This gives you a suboptimal battle-field where stressed-out cells are constantly trying to survive, and an additional insult, like a viral infection, hits you that much harder. To protect yourself from this, it's important to understand your glutathione pathway so you know what your risks are when it comes to inflammation and cellular health.

Methylation

One of the most important but misunderstood cellular processes in your body is methylation. This is when methyl groups are sent to toxins to bind to them, make them water-soluble, and help you remove them. This is important when it comes to inflammation. Now that we know toxins are in the system, now that we know they're causing problems, how do we deal with the inflammation being caused? Through methylation.

The misunderstanding has been knowing how you rank. We know the MTHFR gene is much studied and talked about in medical circles in terms of understanding methylation, but it doesn't end there. There's a whole system. And having one poor gene or one strong gene doesn't mean you're doing a good job or a bad job. You must be able to interpret the entire pathway to get to your net result. This is where our interpretation has moved away from a singular gene-by-gene interpretation toward a system-based interpretation, where we look at the entire methylation process from beginning to end. Only then can we tell you where you rank and how well you're doing with this process, and therefore how you need to intervene with lifestyle, diet, and environmental change. This is where interpretation needs to move beyond the siloed approach to a functional approach. We have done this by understanding the biochemistry of methylation and mapping the genes to their biochemistry. And it's through that understanding that we can know your net result, how you deal with inflammation, and what you should be doing with your environment, lifestyle, and nutrition to mitigate any problems.

Oxidation

We think of toxicity and toxins as something coming in from the outside, but we also create them internally. Our cells produce oxidants and free radicals that enter our bloodstream and cause the same inflammation and harm that the external toxins cause.

How does this happen? The cell's job is to create energy and stay alive. They take in nutrition from your food and oxygen from your breath, and the cell then converts those sources to energy. In that process you produce oxidants, so that same oxygen that keeps you alive is slowly killing you. That's because the oxidants and free radicals in your system that are produced by this process cause inflammation.

Why is this a problem for some people, but not for others? Our genetic makeup, and how we clear these oxidants at the cellular level, is different for all of us. If you take the person who has the best clearance and the person who has the worst, they could be doing the exact same thing with different levels of stress on their cells.

Where does that stress come from? Something as simple as cardiovascular exercise, which you think is good for you, and is probably good for your heart, may be leading to additional oxidation from this process of taking in more oxygen and converting it into fuel, which then leads to more oxidants. The person who can't clear them is going to have a lot more of it in their bloodstream, causing inflammation and wreaking havoc. Therefore, it's important to understand how you deal with mitochondrial clearance at the genetic level so you know what lifestyle, environmental, and nutrition choices to make.

Aging

When we think about cellular inflammation—cellular damage—that load on our cells, the major outcome that we all want to avoid is aging. In terms of the here and now, yes, let's boost our immunity and detox systems so we can be healthier. But if we look further ahead, we can see what causes aging.

Aging is damage that's being done to the DNA. Externally it's that sagging skin, those wrinkles, that white hair. If we only focus on what's happening on the outside, all we can do is continue masking the white hairs and sagging skin and the wrinkles, but if we look inside and understand why aging even happens, we can move toward dealing with the root cause of aging—cellular health, mitochondrial support, the influence of external toxins, all the things that lead to inflammation, that lead to cellular damage, that lead to DNA damage. Again, our ability to cope is different for each of us, and by understanding your genetics you'll understand your personal risk for this load and what you need to do to prevent the aging issue that you're now masking on the outside.

Here are my own test results for the genes covered in this section:

Gene Tested	CYP2R1	VDBP/GC	VDR	MTHFR	SHMT1	MTRR	GSTP1
Result	AG	CC	CT	CC	GG	GG	AA

Gene Tested	MTR	FYT	SLC23A1	SOD2	GSTT1 (copies)	GSTM1 (copies)	GPX
Result	AG	GG	GG	CC	1	0	CC

Here's how my genes influence my inflammation, immunity, and detox profile:

My ability to activate, transport, and uptake vitamin D is suboptimal. Many functional genes influence my ability to absorb, transport, and activate vitamin D. This ultimately impacts the efficiency with which my body can use vitamin D to perform important functions related to anti-inflammation and immunity.

My cellular response to inflammation via the methylation cycle is suboptimal. This means I am more likely to experience an increased severity in length and symptoms of viral or bacterial infections, such as cytokine storms.

The way my body uses glutathionization to remove toxins such as free radicals, heavy metals, estrogen metabolites, mold, pollution, smoke, chemicals, pesticides, and other environmental agents is suboptimal. Because of this, I am more likely to experience a severe response to a bacterial or viral infection, and I am also more likely to take longer to recover from an infection.

How my body uses antioxidation pathways to remove toxins such as free radicals is considered optimal. This means my body deals with oxidants in an efficient manner and reduces their negative impact on my immune system, aging, and other health outcomes. As a result, I am more likely to recover quickly from a bacterial or viral infection.

In the next section, I'll go into more depth about the genes that influence antioxidation, glutathionization, methylation, and vitamin D.

A Deep Dive into the Gene Pool

When he was doing research for his book *The Blue Zones*, Dan Buettner traveled the globe to uncover the best strategies for longevity found in the places in the world where higher percentages of people enjoy remarkably long, full lives. When he wrote the book, he disclosed the strategies he discovered, blending the unique lifestyle formulas with the latest scientific findings to inspire easy, lasting change that could add years to people's lives. As I read the book, I wondered how anyone could *not* be inspired to learn about a 94-year-old farmer and self-confessed "ladies' man" in Costa Rica, a 102-year-old grandmother in Okinawa, and a 102-year-old Sardinian who hikes at least six miles a day. I know I was, and I still am!

In fact, Dan's research, along with that of many others, has inspired me to dive deeper and deeper into the science that underpins how we can combat inflammation, build immunity, and bolster our detoxification system. As I said earlier, the answer lies not in looking at individual genes but in looking at complex gene pathways, systems that work together in a whole-body approach to healthy living, and making choices about the nutrition, environment, and lifestyle loads we put upon those genes.

To recap, we are inundated by toxins every day—from internal and external sources alike—that cause inflammation, put a burden on our immune system and detoxification system, and make us susceptible to illness. Everything we process, from the food we eat to the air we breathe, produces toxins. These toxins include internal wastes like excess hormones and metabolic waste, and external toxins like pollutants, synthetic chemicals, heavy metals, and processed foods. All of it negatively impacts our health.

To protect ourselves from this daily barrage, it is critical that we understand our genetic profile so we can know how best to take care of ourselves. Think about it: you wouldn't wear a parka in 115-degree desert heat, and you wouldn't wear a bikini in 40-degrees-below-zero arctic cold. It's the same thing with inflammation, immunity, and detox.

Without understanding your body's ability to purify itself, your entire body can become "choked" with toxins and other poisons that contribute to heavy metal toxicity, chronic fatigue syndrome, and neurodegenerative disease *and* leave your systems weakened and more prone to sickness and infection.

So let's look a little deeper at the genetic pathways that are responsible for how we handle inflammation, immunity, and detox-ification. For context, I'll share how my own genetic pathways help and hurt my ability to handle these all-important tasks.

Antioxidation

Reactive oxygen species (ROS), also known as oxidants or free radicals, are an example of internal inflammatory agents. At a certain level, free radicals are beneficial for cellular function. However, during infections, the antioxidant defense system of the cell can become overwhelmed. As a result, the cell is exposed to excessive levels of free radicals. Thus, a viral infection loop can occur where a virus infects the cells, causing excess free radical production, and the excessive free radicals make it easier for the virus to replicate.

Maintaining a healthy balance of cellular ROS (free radicals) is referred to as redox homeostasis. A couple of functional genes known as superoxide dismutase 2 (SOD2) and glutathione peroxi-dase (GPX) play important roles in maintaining redox homeostasis.

Another important parameter for viral replication and pathoge-nicity is the availability of host-cell micronutrients. During a viral infection, viruses use the nutrients and machinery that otherwise keep the cell healthy for their own replication. One example of these micronutrients is selenium, which is an essential component of a family of enzymes and proteins known as selenoproteins. GPX is an example of a selenoprotein.

Suboptimal variations in both SOD2 and GPX, coupled with micronutrient insufficiencies of selenium and other important micronutrients and antioxidants, can create a cellular environment that favors viral replication.

In my case, my body does a good job of using antioxidation pathways to remove toxins such as free radicals. This means my body deals with oxidants in an efficient manner and reduces their negative impact on my immune system, aging, and other health outcomes. As a result, I am more likely to recover quickly from a bacterial or viral infection.

I also quickly convert oxidants into hydrogen peroxide via the superoxide dismutase 2 pathway. While this is protective from an oxidant perspective, if you also carry a TT version of your GPX gene in combination with a CC version of your SOD2 gene (I have the CC version but not the TT version), you are more likely to see the graying and whitening of your hair much earlier in life.

The SOD2 gene encodes the SOD2 enzyme, superoxide dismutase 2, which is responsible for removing ROS by converting them into hydrogen peroxide and diatomic oxygen.

I convert hydrogen peroxide quickly into water and diatomic oxygen. If you also have the TT version of the SOD2 gene, you may want to speak to your practitioner about monitoring your hydrogen peroxide levels to ensure you're maintaining appropriate levels.

The GPX gene encodes the GPX enzyme. Glutathione peroxidase is responsible for removing ROS by converting hydrogen peroxide formed by SOD2 into water. I have the CC version of the GPX gene.

I have an optimal version of the SLC23A1 gene (GG), which helps me transport vitamin C throughout the body in an optimal manner. The SLC23A1 gene directs the absorption and tissue distribution of dietary vitamin C. Vitamin C acts as a potent antioxidant and direct scavenger of free radicals. Humans are unable to synthesize vitamin C and must rely solely on dietary sources.

Glutathionization

Glutathionization is one of the most important detoxification and antioxidation mechanisms in your cells. The better your cells are at this process, the better they are at metabolizing and reducing the harmful effects of toxins and oxidants. Conversely, the less optimal your cells are at glutathionization, the more at risk they are for being damaged by toxins and oxidants.

Your GST gene family determines the efficiency of your cellular glutathionization. People with suboptimal variations in their GST family of genes are significantly less able to use glutathione to neutralize excess oxidants and toxins. These people are often much more sensitive to aerosolized toxins and inflammatory agents. They are often more sensitive to strong perfumes, air fresheners, and off-gassing in freshly painted rooms. They also tend to be particularly sensitive to mold.

Unfortunately, the way my body uses glutathionization to remove toxins such as free radicals, heavy metals, estrogen metabolites, mold, pollution, smoke, chemicals, pesticides, and other environmental agents is suboptimal. This means I am more likely to experience a severe response to a bacterial or viral infection, and I am also more likely to take longer to recover from an infection.

My genes are evidence of this. For instance, I carry one copy of the GSTT1 gene. This means I have only an average ability to remove toxins and harmful agents from my body. The GSTT1 and GSTM1 genes influence the efficiency of the GSTT1 and GSTM1 enzymes, respectively. These enzymes are generally responsible for removing free radicals, which can cause mitochondrial and overall cellular damage. Health outcomes associated with poor GSTT1 and GSTM1 functioning include fatigue, tiredness, and lack of energy.

I am missing both copies of the GSTM1 gene; I do not carry this gene in my DNA. As a result, my ability to remove toxins and other harmful substances is significantly reduced.

I carry the optimal version of the GSTP1 gene, which means I am more likely to manage and remove heavy metals from my body, as well as to resist sensory overload when it comes to strong smells and scents. The GSTP1 gene influences the efficiency of the GSTP1 enzyme, which is involved in removing toxins like mold, cigarette smoke, perfumes, and polyaromatic hydrocarbons. Health outcomes associated with a poor GSTP1 result often include migraines and nerve and muscle pain.

Methylation

Viral and bacterial infections can cause several related health outcomes such as cytokine storms, lower respiratory tract distress, acute lung injury, and pneumonia. All of these outcomes have one common characteristic—cellular inflammation.

The purpose of methylation is to reduce inflammation in the body. Having one or two suboptimal or weaker versions of the genes doesn't necessarily mean that your overall cycle is suboptimal. The cycle's overall efficiency is most important, because it can override any individual gene result in this cycle.

My cellular response to inflammation via the methylation cycle is suboptimal. This means I am more likely to experience an increased severity in length and symptoms of viral or bacterial infections, including cytokine storms (dangerous hyperimmune responses).

I am more likely to have optimal MTHFR enzyme function. Note: We evaluate two single nucleotide polymorphisms (SNPs) for the MTHFR gene. Their respective results are cumulative, so it's possible to be optimal for one SNP and not for the other. Being optimal for both (which I am) is the most desirable, while being suboptimal for both is likely to be the most detrimental to your MTHFR function.

Based on my test results, I am more likely to have optimal SHMT1 enzyme function.

I am more likely to have suboptimal MTRR and MTR function.

Since I am more likely to have suboptimal FUT2 enzyme function when it comes to vitamin B_{12} absorption, I take my B_{12} in a sublingual form (dissolved under the tongue).

Note: This version of the FUT2 gene can impact gut microbiome function in a positive manner—if you have this version you should talk to our clinicians to learn more about FUT2 and the gut microbiome.

Vitamin D

Vitamin D technically is not a vitamin. The way that your body makes, transports, and responds to vitamin D makes it more like a hormone. Vitamin D is one of the most important hormones in your body. It is either responsible for or contributes to many critical cellular processes.

Optimal vitamin D levels are needed for optimal functioning of your immune system and for optimal mood and behavior. It even contributes to normalizing your blood pressure and blood sugar and aids in your anti-inflammatory capacity. In addition, vitamin D has been well studied as a co-treatment for pneumonia and moderating the cytokine storms associated with certain infections, including viral infections like COVID-19.

In my case, my ability to activate, transport, and uptake vitamin D is suboptimal.

Many functional genes influence a person's ability to absorb, transport, and activate vitamin D. This ultimately impacts the efficiency with which the body can use vitamin D to perform important functions related to anti-inflammation and immunity.

CYP2R1 is in charge of converting the vitamin D_2 that you absorb from the sun or from plant sources into its active vitamin D_3 form. Because I have the suboptimal version of the CYP2R1 gene, I don't effectively convert vitamin D_2 (ergocalciferol) into vitamin D_3 (cholecalciferol). To counteract that, I take preactivated vitamin D_3 as a supplement. If you're a vegan, seek out synthetic or cultured vitamin D_3 instead of taking vitamin D_2.

The vitamin D binding protein (VDBP), also known as the group control protein (GC), is responsible for transporting vitamin D from its site of activation to its site of action, where vitamin D can bind to the vitamin D receptor and initiate its influence on the body. I carry the optimal version of the VDBP/GC gene. This means I efficiently transport vitamin D in my body.

The VDR gene influences how efficiently vitamin D binds and activates its influence on the body at the receptor site. The VDR transcriptome is strongly correlated to your immune response, hormone production and balance, and even your mood and behavioral patterns. Because I carry the suboptimal version of the VDR gene, I have poor vitamin D binding and activation at the receptor site.

In conclusion, it's critical to know that optimal immunity starts with prevention. The healthier your lifestyle, diet, and environment based on your genetic profile, the stronger your immune system becomes. In general, this means you are less likely to experience severe symptoms from infections and more likely to recover quickly from an infection when you do get one.

Regardless of your genetic profile, with the appropriate personalized interventions you can support the development of a healthy immune system and maintain it throughout your life.

Having said that, I want to give you an idea of what suggestions look like in the context of my own inflammation, immunity, and detox profile.

Glutathionization

Lifestyle

- Increase your intake of fresh citrus fruit.
- Incorporate herbal teas for liver support, such as milk thistle or dandelion root.
- Eat bitter vegetables to increase liver support (bitter melon, cabbage, collard greens, etc.).
- Stay hydrated throughout the day.
- Adopt meditation, mindfulness, and other stress-management practices to reduce stress levels.
- Sweat on a regular basis for toxicant elimination. We suggest at least 20 minutes of physical activity a minimum of three times a week.
- Ensure adequate rest and recovery time between exercises.
- Make optimal, regular sleep a nonnegotiable part of your daily life.
- Ensure your bowel movements are regular and daily for toxicant elimination.
- Minimize exposure to synthetic chemicals in the air, food, and water.
- Ensure a clean environment for living and working.

Habits to Adopt

- Every time you shop for groceries, add citrus fruits, even if it's just a few lemons.

- Cut oranges into wedges and eat a couple for an afternoon snack each day.

- Squeeze fresh lemon juice into a big glass of water each morning. At first, it may strike you as sour, but over time you'll acclimate and enjoy the refreshing start to your day.

- Each morning, turn on a kettle to boil water for tea. This is the starter step to a wonderful habit.

- Ask guests visiting you—at home or at work—if they would like tea. Some cultures do this naturally, but other cultures don't embrace tea as a hospitality habit. It's a great time to start that, right?

- When you arrive home from grocery shopping, wash and store your vegetables so they are ready to cook.

- Always include a bitter vegetable in your evening meal.

Behaviors to Avoid

- Having a diet high in inflammatory foods.

- Consuming large amounts of canned vegetables. They lack the nutrition you seek and are chock-full of sodium.

- Assuming you still dislike the taste of collard greens or broccoli if you haven't tried them recently—tastes change.

- Saying no when you see any of these vegetables on a restaurant menu. Experiment when dining out. You may discover new ways to prepare these healthy heroes.

- Smoking and/or drinking alcohol.

- Spending excessive time in toxic environments such as designated smoking areas, high pollution environments, moldy environments, and areas with high pesticide use (this includes golf courses!).

Supplements

- Detox Optimizer
- NAC

- Milk thistle
- Selenium
- Manganese
- Alpha-lipoic acid
- Vitamin C

Methylation

Lifestyle

- Prioritize vitamin B-rich foods (mainly B_{12}, B_6, B_2, and B_9) found in sustainable fish, organic eggs, organic spinach, beer yeast, and nutritional yeast.
- Cut fast, fried, and sugary foods from your diet.
- Check your home regularly for the presence of mold.
- Buy an air purifier for your home and workplace.
- Build some form of physical activity into your daily calendar.
- Avoid alcohol and smoking—seek out support and accountability if you're looking to quit.

Habits to Adopt

- Portion at least 50 percent of your plate with high-fiber green vegetables rich in vitamins B_9 and B_{12}.
- Add 1 to 2 tablespoons of an organic and/or biodynamic olive oil to your food daily.
- Engage in physical activity at least three times a week.

Behaviors to Avoid

- Spending significant amounts of time in areas high in pollution, smog, mold, or chemicals.
- Living a sedentary lifestyle.

Supplements

- Vitamin B_9—Check your SHMT1 result. If it's the AG or AA version, seek out adenosyl folate (also known as folinic acid) and avoid methyl folate (or 5-MTHF)

- Vitamin B$_{12}$—Check your MTR result. If it's the AG or GG version, seek out adenosyl cobalamin and avoid methyl cobalamin.

- Check your FUT2 result. If it's the AG or GG version, take your B$_{12}$ supplementation as a sublingual tablet.

Vitamin D

Lifestyle

- Ensure you're eating plenty of foods fortified with vitamin D, including dairy or nondairy products, fatty fish, eggs, and meat.

- For vegetarians and vegans, mushrooms provide a good source of vitamin D. However, if your CYP2R1 result is suboptimal, you won't benefit from plant-based vitamin D, since you don't convert it effectively into active vitamin D. Use a synthetic form of vitamin D$_3$ instead.

- Create an outdoor lounge area where you can read, sip tea, or talk on the phone with friends.

- Start an outdoor garden.

- Move a chair or couch in your home (or office) very close to a window that gets direct sunlight.

- Find a friend who wants to take walks outside with you on a regular basis.

Habits to Adopt

- Walk outside every morning for 30 minutes or longer.

- Garden in the afternoon each day for 15 minutes.

- Read outdoors (in your yard or the park) each day.

- Swim in an outdoor pool.

- Wear shorts on any day that's warm enough to do so.

- Take one phone call or meeting standing in front of your window during the day.

Behaviors to Avoid

- Don't work in an office or room that gets only low or no sunlight.
- Avoid careers that require night shifts.

Supplements

- Vitamin D—Talk to your clinician about taking a higher dose than the standard recommendation.
- Split your dose into a morning and afternoon dose if your GC result is suboptimal.
- Take only Vitamin D_3, not D_2, if your CYP2R1 result is suboptimal.

You may notice that I didn't receive or share any suggestions for antioxidation, which is a key part of this section. The reason for that is because my genome is already optimal! I point this out because you should not look at the suggestions I received and think you need to implement them. You need your *own*.

In the final chapter, we will look at longevity—because who doesn't want to live forever!?

Chapter 10

DNA AND LONGEVITY

Curing aging is a hugely important humanitarian goal which would alleviate suffering on the grandest possible scale.

— DR. ANDREW STEELE, COMPUTATIONAL BIOLOGIST, RESEARCH FELLOW AT THE FRANCIS CRICK INSTITUTE IN LONDON, AND AUTHOR OF *AGELESS: THE NEW SCIENCE OF GETTING OLDER WITHOUT GETTING OLD*

Throughout history, people have sought magical ways to restore their youth. One such way, a mythical fountain capable of preserving life, has been a popular legend for centuries. We all know the story of how the Spanish conquistador Ponce de León was said to have searched for the fountain of youth in Florida in the early 1500s. But the quest for immortality was embarked upon much earlier than that.

In the third century, the first emperor of China, Qin Shi Huang, funded an expedition to the East China Sea to find the "elixir of life" that would give him eternal life. Legend has it that Alexander the Great reportedly found a healing "river of paradise" that cured aging as long ago as the fourth century B.C. And in the oldest written story to ever exist, *The Epic of Gilgamesh*, King Gilgamesh, who ruled Sumerian Uruk (modern-day Iraq) in the year 2700 B.C., tried and failed to find a magical plant that would restore his youth. How did Gilgamesh get the idea that defying death was even a possibility? He'd heard about the magic plant from an ancient seer named Utnapishtim, the only human being to survive the Great Flood, who was, afterward, granted immortality.

As evidenced by history and the human struggle, the quest to prevent illness, increase one's vitality, and gain eternal life has always been, and will always be, with us.

Why is this so? Why do we chase a goal of living forever when aging is a natural biological process that occurs in all living creatures? Is this quest the biomedical explorer's version of sailing endlessly in landless seas?

The number one cause of illness, suffering, and death is aging. But it doesn't necessarily have to be that way. With the development of new medicines, procedures, and interventions offering us the possibility to both live longer and to live healthier, why not try for immortality? At the very least, we'll get a lot healthier in the process.

In humans, the speed at which you age depends on several internal and external factors, such as nutrition, lifestyle, physical and mental stress, the environment, and genetics. In fact, variations in your genes can influence how well you manage all the factors that ultimately influence your aging process.

Modern science and technology have improved our ability to slow down and in some cases reverse the biological aging process. However, the most efficient approach to achieving a longer and healthier life is to personalize your approach based on your unique dietary, lifestyle, environmental, and genetic factors.

Once I had my genome tested, analyzed, and interpreted, I was able to learn about my body's ability to access and improve the expression of my longevity gene; recover from physical exercise, infections, and lack of sleep; put on and retain lean muscle mass as I age; fight off free radicals that speed up the aging process; resist cognitive decline and maintain optimal brain health; and ensure optimal bone health.

Short of living forever, that all sounds pretty good, doesn't it? I'm here to tell you that it's just as possible for you to achieve these outcomes as it is for me. And it all starts with getting your genome tested.

Here are my own test results in the area of longevity.

Gene Tested	MTR	MTRR	SHMT1	MTHFR	MAO	COMT	5-HTTLPR	UGT2B17 (copies)
Result	AG	GG	GG	CC	GG	GG	SS	1

Gene Tested	APOE3	AR	FUT2	FOXO3	CYP2R1	SOD2	VDR	CYP17A1
Result	3/3	CC	GG	GT	AG	CC	CT	GG

Gene Tested	VDBP/GC	ADRA2B	TCF7L2	GSTT1 (copies)	GSTM1 (copies)	GSTP1	GPX
Result	CC	ID	TT	1	0	AA	CC

In the next section, I'll go through how my body is genetically equipped for the task of longevity across several systems. In reading it, you will get somewhat of an idea of how your results will read when you get tested, and what those results might mean for you.

Biological Immortality

I always enjoyed watching old reruns of the 1960s television show *Star Trek*. The idea of a diverse and brilliant group of people exploring the universe, seeking out "new life and civilizations," and boldly going "where no man has gone before" filled my fertile mind with fantastical wonder.

But until recently, I had no idea that some version of Spock's Vulcan salute and blessing upon greeting or departing from someone—splitting his fingers into a "V" and saying "Live long and prosper"—is present in all three of the Abrahamic faith traditions, as is some form of the response, "Peace and long life." I also didn't know that the average life span of a Vulcan was 200 years, and that Spock, who prized logic above all else, was a man/Vulcan after my own heart!

We've been expanding our life expectancy for thousands of years. On average we lived to be 19 1,000 years ago and 37 in 1800, but today it's about 78. In the not-too-distant future, the years we'll be able to add to our lives will outpace the time that has elapsed. For example, although 5 years may have passed, we'll have added 10 years to our lives—a net gain. The inventor and futurist Ray Kurzweil, whom we talked about in the chapter on biomedical explorers, believes this and says, "We can now talk about a scenario in which we extend our longevity indefinitely." Ray leans heavily on how the exponential growth of information technology, including microscopic robotic devices that will enter our bloodstreams and overcome disease and aging, will extend our lives. I'm with Ray, although the practicality of advancements will lean just as heavily on human intervention as on information technology.

A few nonhuman species are already capable of biological immortality. The immortal jellyfish, for example, is arguably one of the most intriguing creatures in the ocean. This jellyfish can live indefinitely, unlike any other creature. After growing to its adult stage of life and reproducing, the immortal jellyfish reverts to its juvenile stage and begins life anew. Since it's possible for them to do this as many times as they want, there lies the possibility that they could live forever.

Lobsters, who do not die of aging, are close to biological immortality. Using an enzyme called telomerase, lobsters endlessly repair their telomeres, which are lost when their cells divide. This means they can replace their cells in perpetuity. No zombie cells for lobsters! The only thing keeping lobsters from biological immortality is that they outgrow their shells, become exhausted trying to survive, and fall prey to disease and predators.

Whether it's through information technology, advances in functional genomics and medicine, or a combination of both, biological immortality is an important topic. I anticipate much more research on biological immortality because it can offer groundbreaking insights into human aging and cell behaviors.

In the meantime, using my own longevity genetic test results, let's look at how the body is genetically equipped for the task of longevity across several systems.

Brain Health

Your brain health is a big part of the overall aging process. Cognitive health can remain good for several years after physical decline occurs in the rest of your body. Studies show that maintaining optimal cognitive health is a key factor in increased longevity across global populations.

How do you ensure that you keep your brain as sharp as possible for as long as possible? By understanding not only the physiological but also the mental and emotional aspects of your brain health that are influenced by your genes.

Alzheimer's, Dementia, Cognitive Impairment

Your APOE gene (the version I have is considered normal) plays an important role in the health of your brain. Variations in your APOE gene influence your risk for the depositing of amyloid, which is a mutated protein, in your brain. The increased presence of amyloid in your brain can increase your risk of cognitive disorders like Alzheimer's disease, other types of dementia, and mild cognitive impairment (MCI).

Insulin Resistance

I covered this extensively in the DNA, Diet, and Nutrition chapter, so I'll spare you another lecture. With the version that I have of this gene, I have an increased predisposition toward insulin resistance, which could lead to both type 2 diabetes and cognitive disorders like Alzheimer's or dementia. If you also carry the 3/4 or 4/4 version of the APOE gene, you need to be extra careful of sugar, carbohydrate, and fat intake in your daily diet.

Stress, Resilience, and Aging

Chronic stress is a major contributing factor to the aging process. It is associated with an increased risk of developing obesity, heart disease, mental health disorders, and many other chronic diseases. Importantly, stress is a compounding factor. The older you get, the more stressors you accumulate at a faster rate than the stressors you eliminate.

A person's resilience threshold, or the extent to which they can resist being influenced by stress, is strongly influenced by the versions of functional genes that they carry in their DNA. For instance, I carry the fast versions of my COMT gene and MAO gene. This means I approach stressful situations as a challenge to be overcome, and I don't stop until I've completed the challenge. Sometimes, stressful events can take up my brain space for a longer time than I would expect. COMT and MAO genes influence your ability to move in and out of an emotionally charged state by determining how long neurotransmitters like dopamine and noradrenaline stay active in your brain.

I carry the ID version of the ADRA2B gene. This means I understand and relate to the emotional state of others, but it also means I am more likely to be influenced by their emotional states myself. In addition, I may take on the stress of others, which compounds my own stressors.

Stress adds up over time, for some people more than others. Your ADRA2B gene influences how long you stay in an emotionally charged state (also known as the fight-or-flight response) by determining how long your noradrenaline receptor stays active and ready to bind to noradrenaline.

The version of the 5-HTTLPR gene that I have means I am more likely to become irritated when things aren't going the way I want them to. I can be obsessive over details, and that can consume most of my time. I am also more susceptible to the compounding effects of stress over time.

Sometimes, things that normally don't stress other people out can end up stressing me. That's because the 5-HTTLPR gene influences your body's relationship with serotonin, the neurotransmitter responsible for keeping you in a calm and focused state.

Body

Your body is a biological marvel that is designed to work for as long as it possibly can. Your dietary, lifestyle, and environmental choices influence the efficiency of your body's processes in a significant manner. The extent to which those things impact the longevity of your body depends on the genes you carry in your DNA, and, more important, what you do about it. Once you understand your genomic blueprint, you can identify the minor tweaks you need to make to your daily decisions to create a major positive shift in your body's longevity.

Muscle Building and Retention

Lean muscle mass is an important biomarker of longevity. It allows the body to complete essential movement functions such as walking, running, jumping, bending, lifting, pushing, and crawling. The more lean muscle mass you carry and maintain, the easier these functions become, the longer and more fruitfully you can perform them, and the less risk there is for injury during the performance of these functions.

Your ability to build and retain lean muscle mass is strongly influenced by your hormone profile, which in turn is influenced by functional genes. Specifically, the ability of your cells to bind to and activate androgens, a class of sex hormones, can determine how quickly you are able to see results after starting an exercise protocol.

There are several important genes that can help you understand what your unique hormone profile looks like.

The CYP17A1 gene determines how quickly you make testosterone. The version I have produces an increased amount.

The UGT2B17 gene determines how quickly you get rid of testosterone. I do so at a normal pace.

The AR gene determines how well androgens bind to and activate in your cells. With the version I have, I activate and use testosterone well.

In summary, my overall muscle-building and muscle-retention profile indicates I have an increased ability to put on muscle.

Balding and Hair Thinning

Balding and hair thinning are outcomes associated with increased levels of androgens in your body. Higher androgen levels predispose your hair follicles to a shorter growth phase (the anagen) and a longer resting phase (the telogen). The longer your follicles remain in telogen, the less anchored your hair is to your scalp and the easier it is for your hair to fall out. As a result, androgen-dominant individuals are at the greatest risk of experiencing balding and hair thinning.

As I said earlier, I am androgen dominant. This means I am at increased risk for balding and hair thinning. When I saw "increased risk" in my report I had to laugh. I have no hair on my head at all. That's like a meteorologist saying there's a 50 percent chance of rain during a torrential downpour.

Graying Hair

Graying hair is a natural part of the aging cycle. Pigment follicles in your hair die as you grow older, which leads to less and less color in your hair. However, for some individuals graying hair can occur faster than desired. This is due to increased levels of hydrogen peroxide that are produced during the antioxidation process that occurs in your cells.

There are two important genes that control the two-part oxidation process. Your SOD2 gene creates the enzyme that converts harmful oxidants into hydrogen peroxide. Your GPX gene then produces the enzyme that converts hydrogen peroxide into water and diatomic oxygen. If you produce a lot of hydrogen peroxide but don't convert it at an equal rate into water and oxygen, you are more likely to have graying hair.

The versions of SOD2 and GPX that I have produce and neutralize hydrogen peroxide at a fast rate. However, I have a normal likelihood of getting graying or whitening of my hair earlier in life.

Wrinkles

Your skin is the largest organ of your body. Like every organ, it is susceptible to damage over time. Certain genetic factors can increase your risk of health conditions associated with skin health.

Oxidative stress occurs when the body has an increased presence of oxidants (free radicals), which causes the dermis, or inner layer of your skin, to become less elastic. Over time, this results in the appearance and prevalence of wrinkles in your skin. Oxidants can come from external sources, such as smoking, smog, or pollution, or internal sources, such as excessive cardiovascular exercise or estrogen metabolism.

Functional genes in your DNA—GSTT1, GSTM1, GSTP1, SOD2, and GPX—determine how efficient your body is at removing oxidants before they can cause significant oxidative stress. My versions of those genes are suboptimal. This means I am more likely to have higher levels of toxicants and oxidants due to a suboptimal glutathionization profile. As a result, there is a high likelihood I'll develop wrinkles earlier in life.

Cellulite

Cellulite is the result of uneven fat deposits beneath the skin. The most common areas of cellulite development are on the upper thighs, buttocks, arms, and abdomen. Cellulite occurs at a much higher rate in women than in men due to its association with estrogen. Because of its association with fat storage, an imbalance in estrogen levels can lead to excessive fat storage as a response. Individuals who are estrogen dominant or estrogen balanced are more likely to see cellulite. I am androgen dominant, so I have less of a chance of getting cellulite.

Bone

Bone health is an integral aspect of optimal health and longevity. Healthy bones reduce the risk of serious or debilitating injuries.

Conversely, the mental and psychological trauma that can develop due to loss of movement after a serious bone injury can speed up the aging process, particularly in the later years of life.

As the body ages, bone tissue naturally undergoes several changes in its composition, some of which can inevitably lead to bone health concerns such as osteoporosis. In some people, bone health deteriorates at a faster rate than normal. Factors such as obesity, smoking, alcohol consumption, gender, and genetics play an important role in overall bone health and longevity.

Vitamin D genes control your body's relationship with vitamin D, which is arguably the most important compound related to bone health (alongside vitamin K_2). Beyond your vitamin D, your hormone profile plays an equally important role in determining your bone health development at the onset of puberty and its potentially rapid decline as you get older. For both women and men, decline in sex hormone levels can contribute to an increased risk of osteoporosis later in life.

The CYP2R1 gene determines how well you convert vitamin D that you get from the sun into usable vitamin D. The version I have does not do that very well.

The VDBP/GC gene determines how well you take usable vitamin D to where it needs to go in your body. The version I have does this in an optimal manner.

Finally, the VDR gene determines how well you bind usable vitamin D in your cells. The version I have does not bind and activate vitamin D in an efficient manner.

Biodefense

At The DNA Company, we define *biodefense* as "your body's balance between inflammation and detoxification." Ideally, there is a minimal presence of long-term inflammation with quick and agile detoxification processes. Inflammation occurs in response to infections, exposure to toxins, and poor dietary and lifestyle choices. Detoxification serves to minimize and "clean up" inflammation. Several genes and gene pathways influence these cellular processes.

Here, we consider methylation, antioxidation, glutathionization, and FOX03 genes.

The FOX03 gene is popularly known as the longevity gene. Variations in this gene influence the activity of various potent antioxidation cellular pathways. FOX03 helps initiate DNA repair, kill off mutated or dying cells, respond quickly to inflammation, maintain healthy stem cell production, and attack infectious organisms. Carrying at least one G allele in your FOX03 result greatly increases your potential for longevity by reducing your body's oxidative load. I have one G allele and am more likely to have advanced longevity.

Glutathionization

When it comes to aging optimally, your body needs to be well prepared to guard against attacks from toxins, chemicals, and infections.

Glutathionization is the process through which glutathione, the body's major antioxidant, breaks down toxins and transports them to the liver to be removed from the body. Common toxins include mold, smog, pollution, free radicals, estrogen metabolites, drug by-products, and chemicals. Glutathionization is one of your body's major detoxification and anti-inflammatory processes.

Three genes, GSTT1, GSTM1, and GSTP1, control the efficiency with which your body conducts glutathionization. GSTT1 determines your body's ability to deal with free radicals and recover from fatigue and lack of energy. I am average in this regard. GSTM1 determines your body's ability to deal with toxins, particularly in the gut lining. I have no copies of this gene, so I have a difficult time getting rid of toxins and chemicals that could impact my gut lining. GSTP1 determines your body's ability to deal with chemicals, toxins, and heavy metals. It influences your risk of migraines, brain fog, and headaches due to toxin or chemical exposure. The version I have means that I can't resist the effects of chemicals, heavy metals, and toxins well.

In summary, I carry a suboptimal glutathionization profile. I am at an increased risk of premature aging due to a poor response to oxidative stress. I am more susceptible to exposure from toxins and chemicals around me. I likely struggle with sufficient rest and recovery after periods of exercise. I experience periods of fatigue and lack of energy frequently. When I get sick, I need longer to recover. I experience brain fog, headaches, and migraines, particularly when I am exposed to environmental toxins or if I am significantly physically and/or mentally drained. I have felt all of these things firsthand!

Methylation

Like glutathionization, methylation influences your body's inflammatory response. One of its functions is to remove toxins from your body. Depending on the location where inflammation is occurring in your body, the symptoms you experience can be different. Poor methylation can contribute to (but is not the sole cause of) debilitating migraines, muscle and joint pain, and gut health disorders such as Crohn's disease and irritable bowel syndrome (IBS).

Several genes influence your methylation cycle: MTHFR, SHMT1, MTRR, MTR, and FUT2. It is important to understand that it is not the result of any individual gene but the overall efficiency of the cycle that influences how well your body can fight off debilitating chronic inflammation.

In my case, I am more likely to have optimal MTHFR and SHMT1 enzyme function, but I'm more likely to have suboptimal MTRR, MTR, and FUT2 function.

In summary, I have a suboptimal methylation cycle. I am more likely to have difficulty addressing chronic inflammation throughout my body. I am more likely to experience frequent symptoms such as chronic fatigue, migraines, increased infections, longer recovery times, and episodes of muscle and nerve pain.

Antioxidation

Mitochondrial function is an essential part of a healthy aging process. Your mitochondria are the powerhouses of your cells. Their optimal function is required for your body to complete vital cellular processes.

Oxidants—free radicals—are potent inflammatory agents that can wreak havoc on your mitochondria. Increased levels of oxidants lead to oxidative stress, which can cause mitochondrial dysfunction. Mitochondrial dysfunction can contribute to several health outcomes ranging from fatigue to more serious health conditions. It can also contribute to accelerated aging.

Your SOD2 pathway is designed to convert harmful oxidants into water and regular oxygen in a two-part process. It uses two important enzymes, SOD2 and GPX, whose efficiency is influenced by two important genes of the same name.

The important thing when it comes to this pathway is that the overall pathway must be balanced. It is more beneficial for both of your enzymes to be working at the same speed. If one works faster or slower than the other, the result is a buildup of whatever molecule is being produced at higher levels, which can lead to different outcomes. If your SOD2 enzyme works faster but your GPX enzyme works slower, you'll end up with higher levels of hydrogen peroxide, which can contribute to graying hair earlier in life. Similarly, if your SOD2 enzyme works slower but your GPX enzyme works faster, you may end up with higher levels of oxidants and lower levels of hydrogen peroxide.

The results of my SOD2 and GPX enzyme tests indicate that I have an average antioxidation cycle. I respond to the presence of oxidants in an average manner. As a result, from time to time, particularly in cases of significant mental or physical exertion, I experience an increased period of fatigue, tiredness, or lack of energy that requires me to rest and recover for a longer amount of time. It's hard to do that when you're an entrepreneur like I am, but I'm trying!

Conclusion

Aging optimally, increasing longevity, and extending the time in which you are healthy are critical aspects of optimal health and wellness. When you approach your health and wellness through the personalized approach of functional genomics, you are better equipped to achieve optimal health outcomes.

Don't wait until you're "ready" to take the next step and act now to build a personalized plan that includes digital, group, or personal coaching; dietary recommendations; lifestyle recommendations; and supplement recommendations based on your unique genomic profile.

Do it *now*.

About six years ago, when I was just beginning my journey back to health, I stumbled upon a 10-minute CBC Short Docs episode called *100 and Counting: Secrets to a Long Life*. The episode featured Toronto residents Mohammed Mohyeddin and Ashraf Mohyeddin, 109 and 100 years old, respectively, who had been married for 80 years. Told through the narration of their granddaughter, Samira Mohyeddin, a Toronto-based award-winning journalist, producer, and broadcaster for the CBC, the documentary pondered questions such as How do you stay healthy? How do you stay married? and What are the secrets of a long life?

The promotional blurb from CBC.ca read, "Ashraf is 100 and Mohammed is about to turn 110. They were born in Iran and lived there for 70 years before fleeing to Toronto to escape persecution. Mohammed was a general in the Shah's army; in 1979, he narrowly escaped death at the hands of the new fundamentalist regime with a combination of luck and timing. Canada became Ashraf and Mohammed's new home, and their immigrant legacy is rich. They have a fantastic and successful brood to show for it: 8 children, 20 grandchildren and 11 great-grandchildren—who have all planted roots in Canada."

How could I resist that tease!? And now that I am writing this book, including a chapter on longevity, I want to know how I can find out more about the Mohyeddin family's genetics!

Although Mohammed and Ashraf have both since passed, their story of love, life, and the passage of time gave me a humorous and moving look at the unexpected secrets of a long life. I watched it repeatedly, alternating between laughing and crying. It made me think about my father, made me give my mother an extra hug, and made me grateful that I am helping others prevent and reverse illness, slow down the aging process, and live up to their potential.

It makes me blush to think that I am giving suggestions about how to increase longevity when Mohammed and Ashraf had it figured out already. So I am reminding myself: I don't know their genetics, and I don't know how their lifestyle, nutrition, and environment influenced their genetic expression. I do know mine, however, and I'll share the suggestions that were given to me based on my own genome.

Brain

While you have an otherwise normal APOE profile, your insulin-resistance profile suggests you need to pay close attention to your diet to keep your risk of insulin resistance low. Insulin resistance has been clinically associated with an increased risk of brain-related health concerns such as dementia.

Diet

Carbohydrates are a major focus for you. You'll need to be extra careful about starch (pasta, rice, bread) and sugar consumption. You need to seek out low-carb or no-carb alternatives to starchy carbohydrates and stick to more complex carbohydrates such as sweet potatoes and nuts. You should eat your carbohydrates during the morning and afternoon and skip them for dinner.

A healthy diet focuses on lots of leafy green vegetables (think kale, Swiss chard, and spinach), lean sources of proteins (fatty fish, turkey, minimal red meat), healthy sources of fats (such as avocados and olives), and complex carbohydrates (like sweet potatoes and nuts).

Lifestyle

Engage in brain-boosting activities such as learning and speaking a foreign language or playing chess, sudoku, and other logic-based activities to keep your mind sharp throughout your life.

Stress

Food may play an important role in helping you manage, mitigate, or reduce your overall stress response. However, it also carries the possibility of becoming a coping mechanism, which can lead to bad habits and an increased risk of cognitive decline.

Diet

Top foods to reduce stress: chamomile or lavender tea, warm soups or stews, dark chocolate (a modest amount)

Identify your favorite comfort foods, then focus on creating healthier alternatives to satisfy your cravings during stressful moments.

For example, if mac and cheese is your thing, choose to make butternut squash mac and cheese instead. For ice cream lovers, buy a powerful blender and start using frozen bananas as your ice cream base instead.

Have a cup of herbal tea in the evening just after dinner. Treat this moment as yours: reflect on your day and the things for which you are grateful.

Lifestyle

Develop a regular practice of breath work and/or meditation. This can be done with the aid of YouTube or a teacher in person or online. Research confirms that regular practice will build better perspective and physical resilience to stressful events.

Another habit that can put into perspective and enable awareness of control is making a list of things that are causing you stress. Common sources of stress include work, family relationships, financial problems, social situations, and body perception.

Once you have a list of what causes you stress, identify what you can realistically do about each matter. Following this, create a plan to implement what can be done. To ensure that your plan translates from paper into action, create reminders for yourself: pencil it into your calendar, make a reminder on your phone, or put a sticky note where you'll always see it.

Body

Muscle building will be easier for you than for most other individuals.

Concentrate on compound exercises (bench presses, squats, deadlifts) for maximum output with minimum input as a sustainable workout regimen.

Ensure adequate rest and recovery between workouts.

Hair

Diet

Incorporate fenugreek, which is used mostly in Southeast Asian and Mediterranean cuisines and can also be consumed as a tea. In medicinal quantities, it is a blocker of DHT. Excess DHT levels are a strong contributing factor to hair thinning and male pattern balding.

Incorporate lycopene, which is a compound from the family of carotenoids that gives many fruits and vegetables their bright red color. It is a powerful antioxidant as well as a modulator of DHT levels. Lycopene can be found in high levels in cooked tomatoes, watermelon, and pink grapefruit.

Lifestyle

Be mindful of the hair-cleaning products you use and ensure they do not contain hormone disruptors. Also consider scalp massages and other practices that improve blood flow.

Graying

My results suggest I am not more likely to have graying hair early in my life. However, if I am looking to slow it down even when I am older, consider the following recommendations.

Follow a regular exercise schedule. It helps slow down the aging process because exercise stimulates catalase and glutathione peroxidase production. These two enzymes quickly break down hydrogen peroxide, which is the major cause of graying hair.

Building a regular exercise schedule can be challenging at first, so it helps to keep reminders of why it's so important clearly visible throughout the day. Try changing your laptop or phone screen to a picture or words that keep your motivation up. Remember, starting a habit is always the hardest part; it gets easier from there!

Wrinkles

A sustainable long-term antiwrinkle plan depends on making the right choices when it comes to battling oxidative stress.

Lifestyle

Get enough sleep—this point can't be stressed enough, pun intended. Sleep is your most powerful antiaging tool because all the important processes in your body, like glutathionization and antioxidation, happen frequently when you are engaged in deep, restful sleep.

Another point to highlight is hydration. Ensuring that your body is hydrated is important not only to the appearance of the skin but also to its ability to function and repair itself, maintain elasticity, and keep itself clean.

Download a bedtime reminder on your phone that can lock your screen with a complicated password after a certain time at night so you are not tempted to keep using it late into the night.

First thing in the morning, drink a large glass of filtered water. To remind yourself, this glass can be filled before you go to bed and kept on your nightstand.

Diet

Incorporate antioxidant-rich foods into your diet—blueberries, cacao, matcha green tea with a squeeze of lemon, green peppers, and goji berries. These are just some examples of superfoods chock-full of antioxidants and other stress-fighting compounds that can reduce the level of oxidants in your body that contribute to oxidative stress.

You can also work with a food expert to review your diet and ensure you are getting ideal amounts of vitamin C, vitamin A, B vitamins, zinc, collagen, and healthy oils.

Cellulite

I am less likely to develop cellulite based on my genomic results. If I still struggle with cellulite, I can seek out a licensed practitioner who focuses on hormone balance.

There is a lot of shame and stigma associated with cellulite, and consequently, a lot of pressure to either not get it or to get rid of it. Cellulite is common and not something that per se needs to be treated. Remember, most over-the-counter "miracle" treatments aren't designed to treat the root cause of cellulite.

Bones

Based on my results, I am more likely to have chronically low vitamin D levels, which could impact my overall bone health and longevity. The recommendations below are important, but not the end of the story. I need to work with a licensed practitioner to understand how my hormones impact my bone health.

Supplements

Talk to your practitioner about assessing your vitamin D level and if you should be taking a daily vitamin D supplement. If you do not consume animal products, you can take a synthetic, algae-based, or culture-based form of vitamin D_3.

Ensure your vitamin D_3 is appropriately coupled with vitamin K_2. Vitamin K_2 is essential for bone health as well as a buffer against cardiovascular consequences of excessive vitamin D_3.

Lastly, work with a health care practitioner to evaluate your diet for minerals that are essential to healthy bones. Deficiencies can be addressed through diet or supplementation.

Lifestyle

Get outside often—even if you can't convert vitamin D effectively due to poor genetics, simply exposing your skin to the sun can activate several important processes in your body that contribute to improved mood and cellular function associated with increased vitamin D levels.

Incorporate weight-bearing activities—bones live by the mantra of "use it or lose it." Bones that do not have healthy "stresses" on them do not stay strong. "Stress" your bones by incorporating a weight resistance-training program. Speak with a personal trainer or physiotherapist to create an appropriate program.

Whenever possible, take your virtual meetings outside on the porch, in the backyard, or during a stroll when the weather permits.

Biodefense

My results suggest I could benefit from targeted improvement in important cellular processes that protect my body from infections, inflammation, and aging in general.

Vitamin B_9 (folate) and vitamin B_{12} (cobalamin) are essential to an optimal methylation cycle. Incorporate high-folate foods like spinach, asparagus, and beets into your diet. Incorporate foods high in Vitamin B_{12} such as organ meats, fatty fish, milk, and eggs into your diet. If you are a vegan, source a synthetic, cultured, or algae-based form of vitamin B_{12}.

When considering supplementation, work with your practitioner and your anti-inflammatory report to understand the best forms of B vitamins for you.

Boosting your glutathione levels requires several strategies.

Cruciferous vegetables like broccoli, kale, cauliflower, and brussels sprouts are chock-full of sulforaphane. They sadly can also be chock-full of toxins and hormone disruptors like herbicides and pesticides. To support better detoxification, consume organic cruciferous vegetables. To make sulforaphane more bioavailable, ideally the vegetable is consumed raw (or lightly steamed) and eaten with mustard or a sprinkle of mustard seed powder.

Secondly, be mindful of vitamin C in your diet and increase it if deficient. Vitamin C does the job of scavenging oxidants, which allows your body to stock up on glutathione for dealing with other toxins.

Finally, selenium-rich foods like clams or Brazil nuts are important components of the glutathionization process.

Antioxidant foods are your friends—dark chocolate, matcha green tea with a squeeze of lemon, goji berries, blueberries, green peppers, and pecans are examples of foods high in antioxidants.

Get into the habit of building meals that support multiple anti-inflammatory and detox systems at once. Combine folate-rich foods with foods high in vitamin C to provide a mega-boost to your body's defense systems. Sauté spinach with green peppers, add orange slices to a kale salad, or stir-fry chicken with steamed broccoli and mustard.

Lifestyle

Sleep is a recurring theme in our recommendations. So many of the body's healing, rest, and recovery processes occur when you enter a state of deep sleep. When you fall asleep is just as important as how many hours you sleep; seven hours from 10 P.M. to 5 A.M. is much more effective for the body than seven hours from 2 A.M. to 9 A.M. Get more sleep at the right time!

CONCLUSION

You must be an active participant in your own rescue.

— PAT RILEY, PRESIDENT OF THE MIAMI HEAT AND MEMBER OF THE
NBA HALL OF FAME

I was shocked at how little I knew when I began my journey back to health. Genes, cells, hormones, enzymes, proteins, chromosomes, DNA, alleles, variations, methylation, single nucleotide polymorphisms, and more all blended like a primordial soup in my mind. It was overwhelming.

What's more, I was taken aback by learning about the impact my lifestyle, nutrition, and environment were having on all that stuff. That's what I called it: stuff. How else do you refer to it when you can't differentiate one thing from another?

After I stayed with it and began to understand how my biological systems came together, I realized what I had inside of me was a blueprint for living. An elegant and personalized instruction manual that could help me not only get better but also reverse illness, slow down the aging process, and live with the highest possible performance.

All of that has happened for me, and I want it to happen for you.

I encourage everyone, regardless of their age, to go back to science class. Learn about your cells—the basic building blocks of all living things. Human cells are too tiny to see with the naked eye, but your body is made of 200 different cell types, and between 30 trillion and 100 trillion in total. Each type of cell is specialized to perform a particular function, sometimes by itself, but usually by forming a tissue. Different tissues then come together and form specific organs, with each organ acting like a factory in which every type of cell has its own job.

For example, red blood cells, among other functions, carry the oxygen we breathe around our body. White blood cells are critical components of our immune system. And so on for stem cells, muscle cells, nerve cells, bone cells, and the rest of the 200 types of cells.

Don't stop there. Learn about genes and hormones and enzymes and everything else we've talked about in this book. You've got the power to be a better version of yourself. Take it! And don't do it alone. Get your DNA tested and interpreted so you have the data you need to make decisions. Put together a team of clinicians, nutritionists, and exercise physiologists to help you understand what you need to do, and how, and when. This is how you'll unlock the secrets of your DNA and put them to use to prevent and reverse illness, slow the aging process, and optimize your performance.

This is the DNA way.

ADDENDUM: FREQUENTLY ASKED QUESTIONS

What is a gene?

A gene is a short section of DNA. Our genes contain instructions that tell our cells to make molecules called proteins. Proteins perform various functions in our body to keep us healthy. Each gene carries instructions that determine our features, such as eye color, hair color, and height. There are different versions of genes for each feature. For example, one version (a variant) of a gene for eye color contains instructions for blue eyes, another type contains instructions for brown eyes.

What are genes made of?

Hidden inside almost every cell in your body is a chemical called deoxyribonucleic acid (DNA). DNA is made up of millions of small chemicals called bases. The chemicals come in four types: A, C, T, and G. A gene is a section of DNA made up of a sequence of As, Cs, Ts, and Gs. Our genes are so tiny that we have around 20,000 of them inside every cell in our body. Human genes vary in size from a few hundred bases to more than a million bases. Our entire sequence of genes and bases is called our genome.

What is a chromosome?

A chromosome is a tightly wound coil of DNA. Chromosomes are found inside our cells. Such tight packing allows the DNA to fit inside a tiny cell. We have 23 pairs of chromosomes in each cell, for a total of 46.

What do our genes do?

Each gene contains instructions that tell our cells to make proteins. Proteins perform all sorts of different tasks in our cells such as making eye pigments, powering muscles, and attacking invading bacteria. For example, some cells use genes that contain instructions to make a protein called keratin. Keratin proteins link together in our body to make things like our hair and fingernails.

Where do our genes come from?

Have you ever wondered why you have the same eye color as your dad or the same hair color as your mom? It's because we inherit our genes from our parents. We get half from our mom and half from our dad. When we inherit genes from our parents, we get two versions of each gene, one from our mom and one from our dad. For example, we'll get two versions of the genes that contain instructions for eye color. Some versions of genes are more dominant than others; if we get blue-eye genes from Mom and brown-eye genes from Dad, we will have brown eyes because brown-eye genes are dominant.

If we inherit all our genes from our parents, why aren't we exactly like our siblings?

The reason we're not identical to our siblings is because our mom and dad have two versions of each gene, one from each of their parents. When they pass their genes on to us, they only pass on one of these versions, and it is completely random which one it will be. For example, if our mom has genes for both brown eyes and blue eyes, she could pass the blue ones on to one sibling and the brown ones on to another.

How do genes affect our health?

Our genes are the instruction manual that makes our body work. Sometimes, one or a few bases of the DNA in a gene can vary between people. This is called a variant. A variant means the gene has instructions slightly different from the usual version. Occasionally, this may cause the gene to give cells different instructions for making a protein, so the protein works differently. Luckily most gene variants have no effect on health. But a few variants do affect proteins that do important things in the body, and then we can become ill.

What are genetic conditions?

Genetic conditions are diseases we develop when we inherit a variant in a gene from our parents. As a result, genetic conditions usually occur in families. Scientists have identified more than 10,000 genetic conditions. One genetic condition is called sickle cell anemia. People with this illness have a variant in the genes that contain instructions to make hemoglobin proteins. Hemoglobin helps our red blood cells carry oxygen around our body. These sickle cell hemoglobin genes cause red blood cells to be the wrong shape, making it hard for them to carry oxygen around the body. Not all gene variants cause a genetic condition. Many variants seem to have no effect at all, while others may increase our risk of developing a disease.

What genes cause what common conditions?

Scientists are looking for gene variants that can increase our risk of developing illnesses like diabetes, Alzheimer's, and cancer. It's a tough job, as a lot of illnesses can develop in a very complicated way with lots of different genes involved, and they are also affected by environmental, lifestyle, and nutritional factors like how much we exercise, what we eat, or if we smoke. Rarely, there are people who are particularly at risk of developing breast cancer because they carry some gene variants. Some of these genes have been identified, and it is now possible to look at people's genes to see if they are at risk of developing breast cancer. This can save lives.

How do our environment, lifestyle, and nutrition affect us?

Our characteristics are affected by our environment, lifestyle, and nutrition as well as our genes. For example, we may inherit genes from our parents that should make us tall, but if we have a poor diet growing up, our growth could be stunted. To try and understand how much environment, lifestyle, and nutrition factors can impact us, scientists study identical twins. Identical twins have the same genes, so any differences in personality, health, and ability are caused by differences in where and how they live and what they eat.

Why do scientists study genes?

Scientists have made huge breakthroughs in genetic research over the last few years, learning more and more about our genes and how they make our bodies work. Scientists examine our genes to work out family relationships, trace our ancestors, and find genes involved in illnesses. This gives them the tools to come up with better ways to keep us healthy. A big breakthrough in genetic research came in 2003, with the full sequencing of the Human Genome Project.

What was the Human Genome Project?

The Human Genome Project was an international research study to try and understand our entire genetic code—the complete instruction manual for how our bodies work. Thousands of scientists all over the world worked for over 10 years to read every instruction inside every gene of a group of volunteers and put together a picture of the average human genome. They discovered we have around 20,000 genes in almost every cell in our bodies. Most genes are the same in all people, but a small number of genes, less than 1 percent, are slightly different between people. These small differences contribute to our unique features. Our new understanding of the human genome is leading to many advances in how we treat illness and disease.

How about personalized medicine?

Soon everyone could have their genes read. A doctor might use the information to give us specific medicines tailored for our genes. Currently, many medicines are "one-size-fits-all," but they don't work the same way for everyone. Some people respond well to a medicine, some may not respond at all, and others experience bad side effects. Scientists are learning how differences in our genes affect our reactions to medicines. These genetic differences will help doctors predict which medicines will work for us so they can prescribe personalized treatments.

GLOSSARY

allele

An allele is the version of the gene that is present. Each person has two alleles for each gene, one from each parent. If the alleles of a gene are the same, the person is homozygous for the gene. If the alleles are different, the person is heterozygous for the gene.

chromosome

DNA is packaged into small units called chromosomes. A chromosome contains a single long piece of DNA with many different genes. Every human cell contains 23 pairs of chromosomes. There are 22 pairs of numbered chromosomes, called autosomes, and one pair of sex chromosomes, which can be XX or XY. Each pair contains two chromosomes, one from each parent, which means that children get half of their chromosomes from their mother and half from their father.

copy number variation (CNV)

A copy number variation is when the number of copies of a gene or other section of DNA is different between people.

DNA

Deoxyribonucleic acid (DNA) contains the genetic instructions for all living things. DNA is made up of two strands that wind around each other like a twisting ladder (a shape called a *double helix*). A DNA strand has four different bases arranged in different orders. These bases are T (thymine), A (adenine), C (cytosine), and

G (guanine). DNA is "read" by the order of the bases, that is by the order of the Ts, Cs, Gs, and As. The specific order, or sequence, of these bases determines the exact information carried in each gene (for example, instructions for making a specific protein). DNA has the same structure in every gene and in almost all living things.

DNA methylation

DNA methylation is a chemical addition to a piece of DNA that turns it on or off.

DNA mutation

A mutation is a change in a DNA sequence. DNA mutations in a gene can change what protein is made. Mutations present in the eggs and sperm (germline mutations) can be passed on from parent to child, while mutations that occur in body cells (somatic mutations) cannot be inherited.

dominant

Dominant diseases can be caused by only one copy of a gene with a DNA mutation. If one parent has a genetic disease, each child has a 50 percent chance of inheriting the mutated gene.

environmental factors

Environmental factors can include exposures related to where we live as well as behaviors such as smoking and exercise and cultural factors such as the foods that we eat.

epigenetics

Epigenetics is the study of changes in phenotype caused by something other than changes in the underlying DNA sequence (for example, DNA methylation).

gene

A gene is a part of DNA that carries the information needed to make a protein. People inherit one copy of each gene from their mother and one copy from their father. The genes that a person inherits from his or her parents can determine many things. For example, genes affect what a person will look like and whether the person might have certain diseases.

gene expression

Gene expression refers to the process of making proteins using the instructions from genes. Changes in gene expression can affect how much of a protein is made, as well as when the protein is made.

genomics

Genomics refers to the study of all of the genetic material in an organism.

genotype

The genotype of a person is her or his genetic makeup. It can also refer to the alleles that a person has for a specific gene.

metabolites

Metabolites are the chemicals that are produced by the cells in the body when they break down sugars, fats, and proteins to make energy.

phenotype

Phenotype is how a person looks (on the outside and inside the body) due to his or her genes and the environment (for example, having a certain eye color, being a specific blood type, or being a certain height). Phenotype also can refer to how a person's body functions—for example, whether he or she has a certain disease.

protein

A protein is made up of building blocks called amino acids. The main role of DNA is to act as the instructions for making proteins. Proteins make up most of the structures in our bodies and perform most of life's functions. For example, proteins make up hair and skin. Proteins in our eyes change shape in response to light so we can see. Proteins in our bodies break down food. Proteins are made in cells and are the major parts of cells, which are the vital working units of all living things.

recessive

For recessive diseases, both copies of a gene must have the DNA mutation for a person to have one of these diseases. If both parents have one copy of the mutated gene, each child has a 25 percent chance of having the disease, even though neither parent has it. In such cases, each parent is called a carrier of the disease. They can pass the disease on to their children, but do not have the disease themselves.

single nucleotide polymorphism (SNP)

Single nucleotide polymorphisms are changes at a single DNA base that are present among at least 1 percent of people in at least one population. For example, at a given DNA location, some people will have one base (e.g., adenine), while other people will have a different base (e.g., guanine). The SNP that is more common among a given group of people is called the major allele and the one that is less common is called the minor allele.

BIBLIOGRAPHY

Atkin, Ross. "2012 London Olympics: Don't blink or you'll miss the speeding objects." *The Christian Science Monitor*, August 1, 2012.

Basaraba, Sharon. "A Guide to Longevity Throughout History: Increases in Life Span from Prehistory Through the Modern Era." *Verywell Health*, April 23, 2020. https://www.verywellhealth.com/longevity-throughout-history-2224054.

Buttorff, C., Ruder, T., and Bauman, M. *Multiple Chronic Conditions in the United States*. Santa Monica, CA: Rand Corp., 2017, https://www.rand.org/content/dam/rand/pubs/tools/TL200/TL221/RAND_TL221.pdf.

Chopra, Deepak. *Return of the Rishi: A Doctor's Story of Spiritual Transformation and Ayurvedic Healing*. Boston: Houghton Mifflin Company, 1988.

Centers for Disease Control and Prevention, National Center for Health Statistics. "About Multiple Cause of Death, 1999–2020." CDC WONDER Online Database. Accessed February 21, 2022, https://wonder.cdc.gov/mcd-icd10.html.

Cetlin, Eduardo. "How Do We Get Teens Excited About Science?" *Amgen Foundation*, June 7, 2016. https://www.amgenfoundation.org/News/How-Do-We-Get-Teens-Excited-About-Science.

C. S. Mott Children's Hospital: National Poll on Children's Health, University of Michigan. *Mott Poll Report*, Volume 39, issue 2. August 23, 2021. https://mottpoll.org/sites/default/files/documents/082321_BackToSchool.pdf.

Heineman, Karin. "Ping Pong Balls Break the Sound Barrier," American Institute of Physics: *Inside Science*. July 17, 2013.

Himmelstein, David et al. "Medical Bankruptcy: Still Common Despite the Affordable Care Act." *American Journal of Public Health* 109, no. 3 (March 1, 2019): 431–433.

Mansbach, Adam. *Go the Fu*ck to Sleep*. Brooklyn, NY: Akashic Books, 2011.

Mikulic, Matej. "Prescription drug expenditure in the United States from 1960 to 2020." Statista, July 22, 2022. https://www.statista .com/statistics/184914/prescription-drug-expenditures-in-the-us -since-1960/.

National Health Expenditure Data: Historical. Center for Medicare & Medicaid Services. December 15, 2021. May 5, 2022. https:// www.cms.gov/Research-Statistics-Data-and-Systems/Statistics -Trends-and-Reports/NationalHealthExpendData/National HealthAccountsHistorical.

National Health Expenditure Data: NHE Fact Sheet. Center for Medicare & Medicaid Services. December 15, 2021. May 5, 2022. https://www.cms.gov/Research-Statistics-Data-and-Systems /Statistics-Trends-and-Reports/NationalHealthExpendData/NHE -Fact-Sheet.

National Sleep Foundation: *2006 Sleep in America* (poll), 2006. https://www.sleepfoundation.org/wp-content/uploads/2018/10/ Highlights_facts_06.pdf.

Ornish, Dean. *Dr. Dean Ornish's Program for Reversing Heart Disease*. New York: Random House, 1990.

PBS Newshour. "Inventor Ray Kurzweil Sees Immortality in Our Future," March 24, 2016. https://www.pbs.org/video/inventor -ray-kurzweil-sees-immortality-in-our-future-1466121889/.

Precision Medicine Initiative. The White House Archives. https:// obamawhitehouse.archives.gov/precision-medicine.

Rodriguez, Julia. "CDC Declares Sleep Disorders a Public Health Epidemic." Advanced Sleep Medicine Services, Inc: *The Sleep Blog*, 2018. https://www.sleepdr.com/the-sleep-blog/cdc-declares -sleep-disorders-a-public-health-epidemic/.

Single Care Team. *The Checkup* (blog). https://www.singlecare.com/ blog/news/prescription-drug-statistics/.

Terlizzi EP, Norris T. "Mental health treatment among adults: United States, 2020." *NCHS Data Brief*, no 419. National Center for Health Statistics. 2021. https://stacks.cdc.gov/view/cdc/110593.

Udemy. "Udemy in Depth: 2018 Workplace Distraction Report." https://research.udemy.com/research_report/udemy-depth -2018-workplace-distraction-report/.

Yanping Li et al. "The Impact of Healthy Lifestyle Factors on Life Expectancies in the US Population." *Circulation*, April 30, 2018, https://www.hsph.harvard.edu/news/press-releases/five-healthy-lifestyle-habits/.

Zubrzycki, Jaclyn. "Teens Like Science, Not Science Class, Study Finds." *Education Week*, June 10, 2016, https://www.edweek.org/teaching-learning/teens-like-science-not-science-class-study-finds/2016/06.

INDEX

Lindlahr, Victor, 85
lipoproteins, 137
Lipton, Bruce, 43
liver
    cardiovascular health and metabo-
        lism, 133, 137–138
    cholesterol and, 33–34
    insulin and, 90
lobsters, 190
logic, empathy vs., 62
longevity, 187–206
    actions to take for, 200–206
    antioxidation and, 198–199
    biodefense and, 196–197, 205–206
    biological immortality, 189–190
    body health for, 193–196, 202–205
    brain health for, 191–192, 201–202
    genes related to, 189
    glutathionization and, 197–198
    as goal, 187–189
    lifestyle and, 27–31
    methylation and, 198
low-carbohydrate diets, 94–95
low-density lipoproteins (LDL), 137
low-fat diets, 95–96
lycopene, 203

M

macronutrients, 93–96
male hormones, 151, 158–159
Mansbach, Adam, 122
MAO gene
    diet and nutrition, 88
    and dopamine, 68
    mood and behavior, 44
    testing for, 44
MC4R gene, 89
meat, preparation of, 96
Medical Industry Disruption, 24
meditation, 202
menopause, fitness workouts for, 160
menstruation, fitness workouts and,
    159–160
metabolites, 91, 130, 135, 170, 174, 178,
    197
methylation
    cardiovascular health and, 130–131,
        134, 135, 136, 143
    immunity and, 171–172, 178–179,
        183–184
    longevity and, 198
microbiome, 26, 92–93, 179

micronutrients, 96–99
milk, lactose in, 92
mitochondria
    antioxidation and, 198–199
    detoxification and, 35–36, 39
Mohammed, Mansoor, xvii, xix 12
Mohyeddin family, 200–201
monosaccharides, 94
mood and behavior, 43–83
    addiction, 50–53, 73
    anxiety, 57–58, 75–76
    burnout, 58–59, 76–77
    calm and chaos, 59–65
    depression, 53–54, 74
    diet, nutrition, and effect of, 47
    DNA and multiple influences on,
        overview, 43–45
    emotion and diet, 88, 101
    family, relationships, and effect of,
        45–46
    focus, 65–71
    genes related to, 44
    hypertension and, 140
    irritation and frustration, 62–64, 77–80
    pleasure, overview, 48–50
    procrastination and distraction,
        69–70, 80–81
    sleep and effect of, 47–48
    stress, 54–56, 71–72
    thinking patterns, 64–65, 81–83
    work, career, and effect of, 46–47
motivation, 70–71
MTHFR gene
    cardiovascular health and, 131, 134,
        136
    immunity and, 172, 174, 179
MTR gene
    cardiovascular health and, 131, 134,
        136
    immunity and, 174, 178, 184
    longevity and, 189, 198
MTRR gene
    cardiovascular health and, 131, 134,
        136
    immunity and, 174, 178
muscle. See also exercise
    building and retention, 193–194, 202
    pain/fatigue (myopathy), 138

N

National Health and Nutrition Examina-
    tion Survey (2015–2016), 6

National Sleep Foundation, 110
neurotic tendencies (thinking patterns), 64–65, 81–83
9P21 gene
cardiovascular health and, 131, 134, 135
hormones and fitness, 154
non-celiac gluten and wheat sensitivity, 91
non-REM sleep, 116
noradrenaline, 57, 58, 62, 67, 117, 192
NOS3
cardiovascular health and, 131, 139, 140
hormones and fitness, 154

O

Obama, Barack, 25–27
100 and Counting (documentary), 200–201
opioid pain relievers, 7
Ornish, Dean, 25, 29–30
overeating, 100–101
Ovid (Roman poet), 48
oxidants (free radicals)
antioxidation, 133–136, 176–177, 198–199
creation of, 35
inflammation and oxidation, 172–173
mitochondrial function and, 199
reactive oxygen species (ROS), 176
redox homeostasis, 176
SOD2, GPX, and removal of, 120
toxin removal and, 133

P

pain, addressing, 31
PCSK9 gene, 131, 135, 136
performance optimization, 36–39
personalized medicine, 213
pesticides, 33, 86, 91–92, 95, 104
Ping-Pong (World Fastest Smash Competition), 107
pleasure
addiction and, 50–53
anxiety and stress, 57–58, 75–76
burnout from stress, 58–59, 76–77
coping with stress, 71–72
defined, 49
depression and, 53–54
diet and nutrition affected by, 88
phases of pleasure response, 49–50
sleep and, 118, 125–126
sources of and flip sides of, 48–49
stress, overview, 54–56
polysaccharides, 94
Ponce de León, Juan, 187
postmenopause, fitness workouts for, 160
Precision Medicine Initiative, 25–31
prescription drugs, cost of, 6–7
processed foods, 85
procrastination, 69–70, 80–81
progesterone hormone class, 153
Program for Reversing Heart Disease, 30
protein
amyloid as mutated protein in brain, 191
for brain health, 201
DNA function and, 11
high-protein diets, 96
lipoproteins, 137
micronutrients and, 96–99
selenoproteins, 176
in snacks, 121
vitamin D binding protein (VDBP), 180

Q

Qin Shi Huang, 187

R

rapid eye movement (REM) sleep, 116
reactive oxygen species (ROS), 176. *See also* oxidants
redox homeostasis, 176
relationships, mood and effect on, 45–46
rest and recovery, for fitness, 155–157
retinol/retinyl palmitate, 97
Return of the Rishi (Chopra), 59
reward-based addiction (risk-reward behavior), 51, 52
Riley, Pat, 207

S

saturated fats, 95
Schwarzenegger, Arnold, 146
science education, 19–21
selenoproteins, 176
Selye, Hans, 54–55
senescent cells ("zombie cells"), 35–36
serotonin

V

vascular inflammation, 132, 135, 136, 155. *See also* inflammation
VDBP/GC gene
  diet and nutrition, 98
  immunity and, 174, 180
  sleep and, 112, 114
VDR gene
  diet and nutrition, 93, 97, 98
  immunity and, 174, 180
  longevity and, 189
  sleep and, 112, 114, 115
vegan and vegetarian diets, 95–96
vitamin D binding protein (VDBP), 180
vitamins
  A, 97
  B, 206
  C, 98
  D, 98, 179–181, 184–185, 196, 205

W

weight-bearing exercise, 156, 157, 159, 164, 205
weight management, 148–149
Westheimer, Ruth, 49
Whac-A-Mole metaphor, 3–4
wheat-associated allergy, 91–92
work, mood and effect on, 46–47
World Fastest Smash Competition, 107
wrinkles, 195, 203–204
Wylde, Bryce, xvii

Z

zinc, 99
"zombie cells" (senescent cells), 35–36

ABOUT THE AUTHORS

Kashif Khan is an author, speaker, visionary entrepreneur, and investor based in Toronto who has built, run, and scaled numerous businesses across various industries. He is the founder and CEO of The DNA Company, a digital health company that uses genetic insights to develop genomics-based health management applications that offer patients precision healthcare tailored to their unique biology. Kashif is also biomedical explorer, where he makes health a hobby by constantly seeking out innovation in longevity and wellness to bring under the fold of healthcare.

Rod Thorn is an author, playwright, screenwriter, producer, voice actor, journalist, speaker, strategic advisor, and former communications executive for IBM, Kodak, and PepsiCo. His writing has appeared in *The New York Times, The Wall St. Journal, USA Today, Business Week, Fortune, Forbes,* and other major print and broadcast media outlets. As an advisor to dozens of Fortune 500 CEOs and hundreds of other leaders around the globe, he has been involved in some of the most important developments in business history, the dawning of the Internet, a chess-playing supercomputer, mega-mergers, backbreaking bankruptcies, and cutthroat cola wars among them. He is based in Connecticut.

CONNECT WITH

HAY HOUSE

ONLINE

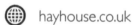 hayhouse.co.uk   **f** @hayhouse

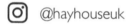 @hayhouseuk   @hayhouseuk

 @hayhouseuk   @hayhouseuk

Find out all about our latest books & card decks • Be the first to know about exclusive discounts • Interact with our authors in live broadcasts • Celebrate the cycle of the seasons with us • Watch free videos from your favourite authors • Connect with like-minded souls

'*The gateways to wisdom and knowledge are always open.*'

Louise Hay